W9-AMA-445

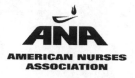
AMERICAN NURSES ASSOCIATION

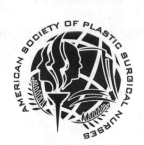

Scope AND **Standards** OF PRACTICE

Plastic Surgery Nursing

2ND EDITION

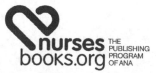
nurses books.org THE PUBLISHING PROGRAM OF ANA

American Nurses Association
Silver Spring, Maryland
2013

The American Society of Plastic Surgical Nurses (ASPSN) and the American Nurses Association (ANA) are national professional associations. This joint ASPSN and ANA publication— *Plastic Surgery Nursing: Scope and Standards of Practice, 2nd Edition*—reflects the thinking of the practice of plastic surgery nursing on various issues and should be reviewed in conjunction with state board of nursing policies and practices. State law, rules, and regulations govern the practice of nursing, while *Plastic Surgery Nursing: Scope and Standards of Practice, 2nd Edition* guides plastic surgery registered nurses in the application of their professional skills and responsibilities.

About the American Society of Plastic Surgical Nurses

The American Society of Plastic Surgical Nurses (ASPSN) is committed to the enhancement of quality nursing care delivered to the patient undergoing plastic and reconstructive surgery and nonsurgical aesthetic procedures. ASPSN promotes high standards of plastic and reconstructive surgical and aesthetic nursing practice and patient care through education, analysis and dissemination of information, and scientific inquiry. For more information: https://aspsn.org/

About the American Nurses Association

The American Nurses Association (ANA) is the only full-service professional organization representing the interests of the nation's 3.1 million registered nurses through its constituent/state nurses associations and its organizational affiliates. The ANA advances the nursing profession by fostering high standards of nursing practice, promoting the rights of nurses in the workplace, projecting a positive and realistic view of nursing, and by lobbying the Congress and regulatory agencies on health care issues affecting nurses and the public.

American Nurses Association
8515 Georgia Avenue, Suite 400
Silver Spring, MD 20910

Published by Nursesbooks.org
The Publishing Program of ANA
1-800-274-4ANA
http://www.Nursingworld.org/

ISBN-13: 978-1-55810-482-2   SAN: 851-3481   06/2013

First printing: June 2013

Contents

Contributors

Scope and Standards Task Force

Sharon Fritzsche, RN, MSN, APRN-BC

Judy Akin, MSN, RN, PHN

Marcia Spear, DNP, ACNP-BC, CWS, CPSN

Patricia M. Terrell, MSN, CPNP, CNOR, CPSN

Jacqueline Frazee, BSN, CNOR, RNFA, CPSN

Claudette J. Heddens, MA, BSN, ARNP, CPSN

Stephanie Dinman, MSN, CRNP, FNP

Christine Brajkovich, BSN, CNOR, RNFA, CPSN

Michelle Rooks, RN

Special thanks to the Clinical Practice Committee Chairman Sharon D. Fritzsche, MSN, RN, APRN-BC, and committee member Judy Akin, MSN, RN, PHN, of the ASPSN for initiating and completing the process of having the ASPSN recognized as a specialty organization by the ANA. Also, a special thanks to the Scope and Standards Task Force members for their work on updating and presenting the new edition of the Scope and Standards of Practice for Plastic Surgery Nursing. The ASPSN would also like to give thanks to Carol J. Bickford, PhD, RN-BC, CPHIMS Senior Policy Fellow, Department of Nursing Practice and Policy, for her guidance and reference in the updates and revisions of the Scope of Practice Statement and revision of the Standards of Practice and Professional Performance for the ASPSN.

American Nurses Association (ANA) Staff

Carol Bickford, PhD, RN-BC, CPHIMS—Content editor

Maureen E. Cones, Esq.—Legal counsel

Yvonne Daley Humes, MSA—Project coordinator

Eric Wurzbacher, BA—Project editor

About the American Nurses Association

The American Nurses Association (ANA) is the only full-service professional organization representing the interests of the nation's 3.1 million registered nurses through its constituent/state nurses associations and its organizational affiliates. The ANA advances the nursing profession by fostering high standards of nursing practice, promoting the rights of nurses in the workplace, projecting a positive and realistic view of nursing, and by lobbying the Congress and regulatory agencies on health care issues affecting nurses and the public.

About the American Society of Plastic Surgical Nurses

The American Society of Plastic Surgical Nurses (ASPSN) is committed to the enhancement of quality nursing care delivered to the patient undergoing plastic and reconstructive surgery and nonsurgical aesthetic procedures. ASPSN promotes high standards of plastic and reconstructive surgical and aesthetic nursing practice and patient care through education, analysis and dissemination of information, and scientific inquiry.

About Nursesbooks.org, The Publishing Program of ANA

Nursesbooks.org publishes books on ANA core issues and programs, including ethics, leadership, quality, specialty practice, advanced practice, and the profession's enduring legacy. Best known for the foundational documents of the profession on nursing ethics, scope and standards of practice, and social policy, Nursesbooks.org is the publisher for the professional, career-oriented nurse, reaching and serving nurse educators, administrators, managers, and researchers as well as staff nurses in the course of their professional development.

Scope of Plastic Surgery Nursing Practice

Definition of Plastic Surgery Nursing

Plastic surgery nursing specializes in the protection, maintenance, safety, and optimization of health and human bodily restoration and repair before, during, and after plastic surgery cosmetic, reconstructive, and nonsurgical aesthetic procedures. This is accomplished through the nursing process, and includes diagnosis and treatment of human response. The plastic surgery nurse collaborates, consults, and serves as a liaison and advocate for individuals, families, communities, and populations, bridging the role of the plastic surgery nurse with that of other professionals to promote optimal patient outcomes for the whole person.

Foundation of Plastic Surgery Nursing Practice

The specialty of plastic surgery has long pioneered surgical techniques and treatment strategies for human body and facial repair, reconstruction, and replacement in cases of congenital diseases, traumatic injuries, and cancer reconstruction. Plastic surgery sites include the skin, breast, trunk, craniomaxillofacial structures, musculoskeletal system, extremities, and external genitalia. Plastic surgery focuses on the care of complex wounds, replants, grafts, flaps, free tissue transfer, use of implantable materials, and the healing process and response. In addition, cosmetic or aesthetic surgery is an essential component of plastic surgery and is used both to improve overall appearance and to optimize the outcome of reconstructive procedures. (American Board of Plastic Surgery [ABPS], 2011). Plastic surgery interventions encompass all ages, from the neonate to the advanced geriatric healthcare consumer. This requires specialized knowledge and treatment to ensure optimal outcomes.

Plastic surgery is the only specialty recognized and supported by the American Board of Medical Specialties (ABMS, 2000) that provides plastic, reconstructive, and aesthetic surgical procedures through board certification for plastic surgery (www.abms.org).

Media coverage to the general public has deluged our society with information about plastic surgery that is often questionable and confusing. Unfortunately, because of extensive media coverage of plastic surgery and increasing demands for aesthetic plastic surgery, procedures are being performed by other medical specialties without proper preparation, recognition, regulation, board certification, or surgical residency experience. This lack of regulation, specialized knowledge, and skill exposes individuals, families, communities, and populations to unnecessary health and safety risks. Both the increasing awareness in our society (accurate and otherwise) of plastic surgery and the ambiguities of cosmetic surgery call for more nursing, consumer, and provider educational interventions by plastic surgery nurses to help clarify misconceptions. Plastic surgery nurses are aware of the health risks associated with plastic surgery procedures and, as members of the interprofessional healthcare team, complement the plastic surgery specialty by a mutual focus on healthcare consumer safety, health maintenance, and ultimate satisfaction and outcomes.

Plastic surgery nursing practice and standards reflect the nursing process, the nursing standards of both the American Nurses Association (ANA, 2010a) and the Association of periOperative Registered Nurses (AORN) standards of perioperative practice, and AORN standards of nursing practice (AORN, 2011). Plastic surgery nursing requires specialized knowledge and skill levels for both the reconstructive and aesthetic aspects of surgical interventions during the consultation, preoperative, operative, and postoperative stages of the plastic surgery procedure process. Through the implementation and maintenance of specialized plastic surgery nursing standards of practice, individuals seeking or requiring plastic surgery intervention will be provided with education, knowledge, and care to ensure optimal surgical safety, protection, and outcomes.

Development of Plastic Surgery Nursing Practice

Plastic surgery nursing opportunities continue to expand as the demand for plastic surgery procedures and treatments grows, primarily in the United States. According to the American Society of Plastic Surgeons (www.asps .org), more than 17 million plastic surgery procedures and treatments were performed in 2009, compared to approximately 1.5 million in 1992. The need for knowledge regarding safety, quality, ethical, and procedural issues will increase as plastic surgery becomes more common in a wide range of surgical environments.

Plastic surgery is an interprofessional specialty. The plastic surgeon's expertise can be utilized by any modality, including but not limited to pediatrics, general surgery, neurosurgery, urology, dermatology, and trauma. Because of the physical and psychological complexities involved in caring for those undergoing plastic surgery, plastic surgery nurses integrate a holistic approach into the plan of care for the plastic surgery healthcare consumer. Plastic surgery nursing skills and knowledge require a strong foundation in the knowledge of pre-, intra-,and postoperative standards and practices; wound healing and wound care; safety and quality; bioethics; psychology; and the application of critical thinking.

In response to the specialized needs of plastic surgery healthcare consumers and the required nursing interventions, 100 surgical nurses convened in 1975 to establish the nonprofit organization called the American Society of Plastic and Reconstructive Surgical Nurses (ASPRSN). In 2001 ASPRSN simplified its name to American Society of Plastic Surgical Nurses (ASPSN). The 100 charter members sought to establish a specialized identity and share the knowledge needed to practice successfully. The mission and philosophy of the ASPSN were founded on principles aimed at improving the quality of nursing care for the healthcare consumer undergoing plastic or reconstructive surgery. The organization is committed to promoting high standards of nursing care and practice through shared knowledge, scientific inquiry, and continuing education, while supporting and encouraging collaborative interaction with clinical practice, administration, research, and academics (www.aspsn.org). The chronology of the development of plastic surgery nursing is summarized below.

Plastic Surgery Nursing: A Chronology

1975   The American Society of Plastic and Reconstructive Surgical Nurses (ASPRSN) held its first national meeting in Toronto, Canada. Sherill Lee Schultz is the first president and founder.

1976   Thirteen local chapters of ASPRSN are established in the United States and Canada.

1980   ASPRSN creates *Plastic Surgical Nursing Journal*.

1980   ASPRSN becomes the 22nd member of the National Federation for Specialty Nursing Organizations.

1984   The plastic surgical nursing bibliography is completed.

1989   The first edition of *Core Curriculum for Plastic and Reconstructive Surgical Nursing* is published.
        The Plastic Surgical Nursing Certification Board (PSNCB) is established.

1991   The first plastic surgical nursing certification examination (CPSN) is given.

1995   ASPRSN establishes a Research Committee to assist ASPRSN nurses with research funds and priorities unique to plastic surgical nursing practice.

1996   The second edition of *Core Curriculum for Plastic and Reconstructive Surgical Nursing* is published.

1998   ASPRSN creates a website: www.aspsn.org.

2001   ASPRSN simplifies its name to the American Society of Plastic Surgical Nurses (ASPSN).

2004   The specialty is recognized and the ASPSN–ANA specialty standards document, *Plastic Surgery Nursing: Scope and Standards of Practice,* is drafted.

2005   *Plastic Surgery Nursing: Scope and Standards of Practice* is published by ANA.

2007   Third edition of *Core Curriculum for Plastic Surgical Nursing* is published.

2010   Task force is initiated to develop an aesthetic nursing certification.

2010   Workgroup is convened to review and revise *Plastic Surgery Nursing: Scope and Standards of Practice.*

Today the ASPSN has more than 1,000 active members working in various nursing environments: surgical facilities, home care, nursing research, outpatient care, hospitals, universities, private practice, medical or medi-spas, and others. Members cover a wide range of educational levels, including associate, bachelor's, master's, and/or doctorate degrees, and have numerous roles, including advanced practice nurses, nurse first-assistant, and nurse educators. ASPSN serves its members through a national structure of local chapters in the United States and Canada (ASPSN, 2010). Through the development of unique plastic surgery knowledge, the plastic surgery nurse can properly respond to and communicate with a multidisciplinary team assigned to any plastic surgery healthcare consumer.

As the field of plastic surgery evolves and incorporates other medical specialties, the climate for plastic surgery nursing requires continual review of related trends, products, and procedures. Current statistical data found on the American Society of Plastic Surgeon's web site (www.asps.org) for 2009, include a 10% increase in breast reconstruction from 2000 to 2009, with tissue expander reconstruction seeing a 12% increase from 2008 to 2009. Breast reduction surgery has increased by 7% from 2000. Tumor removal, including skin cancers, has decreased from 578,161 procedures in 2000 to 487,146 in 2009. Cosmetic surgical procedures have experienced an overall decline since 2000, with a 20% total decrease. Breast augmentation remains the number-one cosmetic procedure, followed by rhinoplasty. With more and more healthcare consumers undergoing bariatric or weight-loss surgical procedures, the number of body contouring procedures (such as buttock lifts, lower body lifts, and thigh and arm lifts) is increasing significantly, and has experienced more than a 50% increase since 2000 (www.asps.org). Minimally invasive procedures have increased 99% since 2000, with Botox showing a 509% increase from 2000; in addition, there has been a significant rise in procedures for dermal fillers and laser resurfacing (www.asps.org). Due to this extraordinary growth, there has been an influx of nurses into this highly challenging arena of plastic surgery practice.

One goal of plastic surgery nursing is to secure the foundation for safety. This is accomplished through stronger regulations, increased education, and awareness among healthcare consumers, families, communities, and populations seeking or requiring plastic surgery-related interventions.

Plastic surgery nurses promote and improve quality of care before, during, and after plastic surgical procedures and treatments to ensure proper health maintenance, safety, and restoration. Plastic surgery nurses determine the specific nursing intervention needed for each individual undergoing a plastic surgical procedure or treatment, in accordance with the nursing process (assessment, diagnosis, outcomes identification, planning, implementation, and evaluation). This nursing specialty continues to develop the knowledge base for evidence-based practice through research into plastic surgery procedures, treatments, and issues.

Healthcare Consumer Population

The plastic surgery nurse interacts with and cares for healthcare consumers who require or desire plastic or reconstructive surgery for enhancement or restoration purposes. The plastic surgery nurse also interacts with wand educates families of plastic surgery healthcare consumers, as well as communities, regarding plastic surgery procedures and issues. The plastic surgery nurse has the special knowledge and skills needed to meet the needs of the healthcare consumer population. The plastic surgery nurse provides care in a variety of settings, age groups, and populations, including neonatal, pediatric, adult, geriatric, general surgery, neurosurgery, advanced wound management, dermatology, burns, cancer, and trauma healthcare consumers.

Healthcare consumers receiving care and education from a plastic surgery nurse need a thorough understanding of procedures, personal expectations, and mutual goal setting in order to achieve maximum satisfaction and health maintenance. Plastic surgery nurses help healthcare consumers to deal with perceived or altered body image, perceived surgical outcomes, fears, and learning needs associated with a surgical intervention. Healthcare consumers undergoing plastic surgery may encounter psychological, emotional, and physical imbalances during the recovery phase. Managing the psychological discord associated with physical alterations requires specialized knowledge and education.

Reconstructive Plastic Surgery Population

Reconstructive plastic surgery procedures are performed on skin, breast, trunk, craniomaxillofacial structures, musculoskeletal system, extremities, and external genitalia. Nurses in reconstructive plastic surgery require specialized knowledge related to complex wounds, replants, grafts, flaps, free tissue transfer, and use of implantable materials for reconstruction or repair due to cancer, trauma, burns, superficial injury, congenital defects, or disease. Plastic surgery nurses help the patient to express psychological, physical, and psychosocial needs in order to regain or rediscover coping strategies and successful interactions with society. Thorough assessment and documentation before, during, and after surgery is essential for proper evaluation of healthcare consumer outcomes.

Aesthetic Plastic Surgery Population

The plastic surgery nurse must possess a thorough knowledge of anatomy, body systems, operative standards, and the psychological aspects of body image and perception. An understanding of the needs and assessment of expectations places the plastic surgery nurse in the forefront as an advocate for the aesthetic healthcare consumer's safety. Aesthetic plastic surgery procedures may be applied to skin, breast, trunk, craniomaxillofacial structures, musculoskeletal system, extremities, and external genitalia. Aesthetic plastic surgery may be performed after reconstructive surgery to improve overall results. Aesthetic surgery includes adjustment, enhancement, and alteration according to each individual healthcare consumer's request and need for plastic surgery intervention. Thorough assessment and documentation before, during, and after surgery is essential for proper evaluation of patient outcomes.

With the development and introduction of new products and technologies, the quest to defy the aging process and enhance beauty continues. According to the 2008 *Plastic Surgery Procedural Statistics* (American Society of Plastic Surgeons, 2009), there has been a steady increase in the number of consumers who have undergone nonsurgical aesthetic procedures, notably injections of botulinum toxin Type A and dermal fillers. This phenomenon has required that healthcare providers adapt to these technical developments to meet the needs of the population, and has led to increased specialization in the area of plastic surgery nursing. In short, plastic surgery nurses require specialized knowledge associated with reconstructive surgical principles to assist in the successful recovery and outcomes of the aesthetic surgery healthcare consumer.

Roles of Plastic Surgery Nurses

Nursing: Scope and Standards of Practice, Second Edition (ANA, 2010a), *Nursing's Social Policy Statement: The Essence of the Profession* (ANA, 2010b), and *Code of Ethics for Nurses with Interpretive Statements* (ANA, 2001) provide the foundation for all registered nurses and their professional practice. The roles of the plastic surgery nurse further derive from the specialty's scope-of-practice statement and specific standards of care, required educational guidelines, and practice environments and settings serving the plastic surgery healthcare consumer. One of the goals of plastic surgery nursing is to reach and educate other nurses and nursing students about plastic surgery issues, procedures, and current trends. Communication and interaction with other nursing specialties about the role of plastic surgery nurses will provide a broader understanding and knowledge base for nursing collaboration. Plastic surgery nurses help build the foundations of knowledge and education for improved outcomes, safety, health maintenance, and health awareness.

General Nursing Role

Registered nurses beginning clinical practice in their first year of licensure are encouraged to gain knowledge and develop skill levels associated with basic medical and surgical principles in preparation for later specialization in plastic surgery nursing. Registered nurses who enter the field of plastic surgery must have a well-rounded knowledge base about a wide variety of healthcare consumer populations. The scope of knowledge required for the plastic surgery nurse varies with the area of practice interest, previous nursing experience, and level of educational preparation. The general-level plastic surgery nurse will progress into a more expert role with experience, training, mentoring, and additional education.

Advanced Practice Role

Advanced practice plastic surgery nursing roles are increasing in response to personal, professional, and societal needs. Nurse practitioner (NP) and clinical nurse specialist (CNS) are two of the roles included in the term *advanced practice*.

Advanced practice registered nurses (APRNs) play a significant role in meeting the needs of the plastic surgery healthcare consumer. APRNs in plastic surgery are valuable in practice because of their ability to use independent judgment in clinical decision-making and to provide skilled, quality, and detailed advanced nursing care across the continuum. An APRN in plastic surgery has the knowledge and training to provide comprehensive health assessments, differential diagnoses, and treatments for plastic surgery healthcare consumers. The APRN in plastic surgery is an advocate for health maintenance, health promotion, and wellness.

Advanced practice registered nurses in plastic surgery serve as resources and consultants to other healthcare disciplines. Legislation has now made prescriptive authority and third-party reimbursement possible for the APRN in the plastic surgery arena. The APRN is instrumental in facilitating and conducting research in plastic surgery and plays a key role in providing continuity of care for the plastic surgery healthcare consumer based on the best evidence. The roles of the APRN in plastic surgery are developing and expanding.

Educator Role

Plastic surgery nurse educators promote educational clarity, standards, knowledge, and safety related to plastic surgery procedures, issues, and outcomes with other nurses, students, healthcare consumers, other providers, and the community. In this document, the plastic surgery registered nurse (RN) in an educator role is referred to as the *plastic surgery nurse educator*.

Even though all nurses are educators in their role of caring for healthcare consumers, a plastic surgery nurse educator is educated at the master's-degree level or higher with a focus on plastic surgery education. A plastic surgery nurse educator requires a strong knowledge base regarding teaching and learning theories, curriculum development, research, test and measurement evaluation methods, critical thinking skills, and quality improvement techniques. Plastic surgery nurse educators also comply with and support state educational requirements to teach at community or university institutions. At the graduate or doctoral level, the plastic surgery nurse educator has the opportunity to facilitate and develop focused education, curriculums, and research in plastic surgery nursing.

A plastic surgery nurse educator conducts a needs assessment to help establish educational requirements in various practice environments and settings. A plastic surgery nurse educator functions as an educator and a liaison between the plastic surgeon or advanced practice registered nurse and the healthcare consumer to help ensure continuity of care, health promotion, and health maintenance. A plastic surgery nurse educator provides an appropriate climate for learning, and ensures that the learners are actively involved in the learning process. The plastic surgery nurse educator collects and analyzes data to evaluate the effectiveness and outcomes of various educational strategies, and, if necessary, provides a revised plan to address shortcomings and problems.

A plastic surgery nurse educator is a member of an interprofessional team, and functions as a consultant, change agent, leader, and resource to other nursing and healthcare disciplines. Plastic surgery nurse educators help to generate research and disseminate findings into education and practice.

A plastic surgery nurse educator, in collaboration with plastic surgery nurses, develops instructions, guidelines, materials, and programs for nurses during nursing school rotations, distance learning experiences, and in various practices, environments, and settings related to plastic surgery. A plastic surgery nurse educator also provides education for local and national communities on plastic surgery and relevant resources.

Specialized Nursing Role

Because the demand for procedures to maintain a youthful appearance and beauty has exploded, the development of new and improved aesthetic nonsurgical technologies, products, and procedures has also grown. This has facilitated the development of the aesthetic nurse role within plastic surgical nursing. With the increasing demand for these procedures, the role of the aesthetic nurse becomes more important in plastic surgery as well as other specialties. The aesthetic nurse has a scope of knowledge more specialized to nonsurgical aesthetic procedures and this population of healthcare consumers than the general plastic surgery nurse, and has undergone additional education and training in anatomy, procedural techniques, products, technologies, assessment, and education specific to the aesthetic nonsurgical healthcare consumer.

The aesthetic nurse must be focused on maintaining the highest standards within the specialty by undergoing continuing education, providing excellent outcomes, and maintaining an unrivaled ethical environment. The aesthetic nurse must always consider the healthcare consumer's specific requests, budget, lifestyle, and expectations. The aesthetic nonsurgical healthcare consumer often hears about new products or procedures via the popular media, so the aesthetic nurse, as a professional, must guide and educate the patient to select an appropriate product, procedure, or technology and make necessary referrals to the physician. As these procedures are out-of-pocket expenses to the individual, the aesthetic nurse has an obligation to recommend and provide only those procedures that are appropriate and to avoid any financial conflict of interest.

Educational Preparation for Plastic Surgery Nursing

Broad experience in surgical duties, sterile technique, and postanesthesia care enhances the ability to build on the skill sets needed for specialty practice. As there are no formal academic educational programs for plastic surgery nursing, plastic surgical nurses must build on the general knowledge and education of their respective nursing programs. The plastic surgery nurse learns plastic surgery fundamentals from professional courses offered by ASPSN, core curriculum materials, mentoring, and seminars and workshops pertaining to plastic surgery education, procedures, and issues. Education, experience, and increased familiarity with plastic surgery procedures and outcomes will increase knowledge and help attain the skill levels needed to care for the plastic surgery healthcare consumer. Due to the complexities of plastic surgery, including psychological and psychosocial factors, plastic surgery nurses require a minimum of two years of experience before seeking certification in plastic surgery nursing.

Minimum Requirements for Plastic Surgery Nursing

- Licensure as a registered nurse within the designated state of practice

- Education:

  - Minimum requirement: Associate's degree from an accredited college of nursing

  - Preferred: Bachelor of science degree in nursing from an accredited college of nursing

- Advanced knowledge in surgical principles, anatomy, and physiology for specified age groups from neonates to older adults

- Advanced knowledge in one or more of the following:

  - Wound care, burns, trauma, cancer-related disfigurements

  - Scar management, body image, health assessment, nutrition

- Continuing education and knowledge of current plastic surgery trends, issues, and procedures

- Certification:

    Plastic surgery nursing certification is available (http://psncb.org/)

- Advanced knowledge and training in anatomy, including muscles and blood vessels, aging, assessment, and technologies (aesthetic role).

Plastic Surgery Nursing Research and Evidence-Based Practice

Evidence-based practice (EBP) is a scholarly and systematic problem-solving paradigm that results in the delivery of high-quality health care. To make the best clinical decisions using EBP, research findings are blended with internal evidence—including practice-generated data, clinical expertise, and healthcare consumer values and preferences—to achieve the best outcomes for individuals, groups, populations, and healthcare systems.

Nursing research and EBP contribute to the body of knowledge and enhance healthcare consumer outcomes. The plastic surgery nurse continually evaluates and applies nursing research findings to promote effective and efficient care and improved outcomes. The plastic surgery nurse works with other members of the healthcare team to identify clinical problems and uses existing evidence to improve practice. Nurses must demonstrate that nursing interventions make a positive difference in the outcomes and health status of plastic surgery healthcare consumers. The plastic surgery nurse uses research findings to decrease practice variations, improve outcomes, and create standards of excellence for care and policies. In addition, the plastic surgery nurse assures that changes made in practice are based on the current evidence and seeks out expert resources to assist with specific steps in EBP. Plastic surgery nurses utilize evidence-based practice to keep abreast of medical knowledge relevant to practice and ensure that they are current and up-to-date on the latest evidence.

Increased demand for aesthetic procedures has resulted in a higher number of plastic surgery nurses undertaking the role of aesthetic nurse. Many aesthetic treatments and procedures that claim to rejuvenate the skin are not supported by good scientific evidence; therefore, the plastic surgery nurse must critically appraise the evidence and utilize only the best evidence to guide practice. In this emerging area of practice, the plastic surgery nurse generates an ongoing, systematic evaluation of long-term outcomes and implements practice changes as appropriate. There is a need for unbiased funding of research in this emerging area of practice, and the plastic surgery nurse is positioned to seek this funding.

EBP undergirds and advances the professional practice of all plastic surgery nurses. Plastic surgery nurses must be able to gain, assess, apply, and integrate new knowledge, as well as the ability to adapt to changing circumstances and environments.

Practice Environments and Settings for the Plastic Surgery Nurse

The plastic surgery nurse provides care for healthcare consumers and their families or caretakers in a variety of settings and locations that include hospitals, outpatient ambulatory surgery centers, office-based surgery centers, private practice, and newly evolving medical spas. The plastic surgery nurse is prepared to educate and provide comprehensive care to healthcare consumers in a safe and regulated environment. The plastic surgery nurse provides competent, ethical, and appropriate nursing care to help improve surgical experiences and outcomes. To determine and implement the plan of care, and to ensure optimal outcomes for the plastic surgery healthcare consumer, the plastic surgery nurse encourages and facilitates consultations, communication, and collaboration with other healthcare team members. As a healthcare provider, the value and benefit of the APRN in plastic surgery practices are widely recognized, and the APRN is being utilized in many or most of the previously mentioned practice settings and locations.

Plastic surgery nurses are also knowledgeable about proper policies, procedures, contracts, and regulations, including those for compliance with the Health Insurance Portability and Accountability Act (HIPAA), in appropriate and designated plastic surgery settings. Plastic surgery nurses know and comply with the requirements for federal, state, local, insurance, and accreditation agency standards, regardless of the area of practice. Plastic surgery nurses help promote safer surgical services for the plastic surgery healthcare consumer. Regulatory factors pertinent to plastic surgery nurses working in any environment may include The Joint Commission (TJC); the Centers for Medicare and Medicaid Services (CMS); Occupational Safety and Health Administration (OSHA) standards for bloodborne pathogens and hazardous waste; the Americans with Disabilities Act; specific hospital rules and regulations; and rules, regulations, and guidelines established by each state board of nursing. All of these ensure public safety. The plastic surgery nurse should also know and address, as appropriate, compliance with the guidelines of the Accreditation Association for Ambulatory Health Care (AAAHC), the AAAHC Institute for Quality Improvement (IQI), the American Association for Accreditation of Ambulatory Surgery Facilities, Inc. (AAAASF), and the U.S. Food and Drug Administration regarding tissue tracking and drug and/or implant recalls.

Hospitals

The plastic surgery nurse working in the hospital environment may care for plastic surgery healthcare consumers in a variety of specialty departments or units. These include, among others, emergency departments; operating rooms; surgical, burn, critical care, and neonatal units; pediatrics; and oncology. Plastic surgery nursing within the hospital environment is multidimensional and includes skills, functions, roles, and responsibilities that evolve from the body of knowledge specific to plastic surgery nursing. The plastic surgery nurse practicing in the hospital environment may provide assessment, analysis, diagnosis, planning, implementation, interventions, outcome identification, and evaluation of healthcare consumers in all age groups whose care requires plastic surgery interventions, procedures, wound care, and other treatments.

Outpatient/Ambulatory Surgery Centers

The plastic surgery nurse working in the outpatient/ambulatory surgery center demonstrates the appropriate skills, knowledge, competencies, and abilities to provide proper and safe nursing care for the plastic surgery healthcare consumer in the preoperative, operative, and postoperative stages of the plastic surgery procedure. The outpatient/ambulatory surgery center must be accredited or certified by the appropriate surgery center accreditation for the state. The plastic surgery nurse working in an outpatient/ambulatory surgery center maintains the plastic surgery nursing standards of practice and standards of professional performance.

Office-Based Surgery Centers

According to ASPS (2009) statistical data, 65% of aesthetic plastic surgery procedures and 46% of reconstructive plastic surgery procedures are performed in a plastic surgeon's office (www.asps.org). This poses risks if the office does not have a properly accredited or regulated surgery facility. Public awareness and understanding of proper accreditation and regulation is needed to provide clarity and guidance when considering plastic surgery. The plastic surgery nurse is aware of the potential confusion surrounding office-based surgery and can be instrumental in providing proper education about accreditation and regulation for other nurses, consumers, and communities.

The role of the plastic surgery nurse in the office-based surgery center includes the consultation, preoperative, postoperative, and follow-up stages of the plastic surgery procedure. The plastic surgery nurse demonstrates the appropriate skills, knowledge, competencies, and abilities to provide proper nursing care for the plastic surgery healthcare consumer. In addition to nursing responsibilities, the office-based plastic surgery nurse may have administrative responsibilities such as staffing, billing, insurance filing, verification and predetermination, as well as budgetary duties including purchasing of medical supplies and equipment.

Assessment, education, planning, and intervention are part of the plastic surgery nurse's role during each stage of a plastic surgery procedure. The plastic surgery nurse helps to improve the quality of care by maintaining standards, including the Standards of Plastic Surgery Nursing, measuring performance, and providing education within the specific office-based surgery center.

Private Practice Settings

The plastic surgery nurse working in a private practice may have responsibilities that include assessing the individual healthcare consumer's needs, developing educational material, assisting physicians or advanced practice plastic surgery nurses, and conducting staff education and in-service and healthcare consumer education. The plastic surgery nurse assesses educational needs and then provides educational material and instruction on the plastic surgery procedure. In addition, there may be management responsibilities such as billing, surgery scheduling, and insurance filing and verification, as well as budgetary duties regarding annual budgets and purchase of medical supplies and equipment.

The plastic surgery nurse also provides preoperative and postoperative counseling regarding technical aspects of the surgical procedure, documented health assessment, pertinent mutual goal planning, and psychosocial assessment and support. Other responsibilities may include sedation, postanesthesia recovery, and assisting with the procedure.

The plastic surgery nurse may provide consumer education about selecting an appropriate plastic surgery facility and provider that will meet the consumer's needs and provide the best outcomes. The plastic surgery nurse in private practice provides follow-up communication and evaluation to ensure quality of care, health maintenance, and proper documentation. The plastic surgery nurse in private practice maintains the plastic surgery nursing standards of practice and standards of professional performance.

Private practice has increasingly become an area for the aesthetic nurse specialty to practice, in collaboration with the physician. In many instances, this aesthetic nurse performs many, if not all, of the nonsurgical aesthetic enhancement procedures within the practice. In this role, the aesthetic nurse will function as counselor, provider, educator, and communicator. The aesthetic nurse maintains the plastic surgery nursing standards of practice and standards of professional and competent performance, as well as high ethical standards.

Medical Spas

New trends and increasing demands for aesthetic procedures have prompted the emergence of *medical spas*; this is a combination of a medical office and a day spa that operates under the supervision of a medical doctor. Medical spas tend to have a more clinical atmosphere than day spas, and can offer a wide range of services and treatments, including hair removal and reduction, injectables (such as botulinum toxin Type A and fillers), chemical peels, microdermabrasion, minor laser treatments, and/or sclerotherapy.

The plastic surgery nurse in the role of aesthetic nurse in these settings incorporates reputable educational preparation, such as workshops, conferences, and industry training, in learning new technologies and products relating to the procedures directly provided. The aesthetic nurse practices for a period of time directly with the supervising physician before practicing independently and is accountable for her or his practice.

Before practicing independently, the aesthetic nurse must gain the skills to assist in the care of the healthcare consumer who desires medical spa treatments and must have specialized advanced training in aesthetic nursing, including facial anatomy, assessment, products, procedures, and technology. The aesthetic nurse must maintain an active, collaborative relationship with the medical doctor of the spa. The aesthetic nurse may utilize protocols that are developed collaboratively with the medical doctor to guide practice. The aesthetic nurse should practice documentation of procedures and postprocedure follow-up. The collaborating physician should perform and document periodic supervision of the nurse's performance, to assure competency. The aesthetic nurse should be responsible for utilizing the best available evidence to guide treatment choices, should provide potential consumers with truthful information, and should not have any conflicts of interest.

Ethics and Advocacy in Plastic Surgery Nursing

Ethics is a fundamental part of nursing. Ethical awareness, judgments, and decisions are founded on a combination of principles, theories, and moral foundations. Nursing ethics are based on care and the actions of caring, to enhance and protect healthcare consumer well-being. Plastic surgery nurses are expected to comply with and promote the ethical ideals, model, code, and principles of the nursing profession. *Code of Ethics for Nurses with Interpretive Statements* (ANA, 2001) is the framework on which plastic surgery nurses base ethical analysis and decision-making, and on which standards are based. The plastic surgery nurse is also an advocate for the healthcare consumer and provides care in a nondiscriminatory and nonjudgmental way. Patient advocacy mandates preservation of autonomy, execution of clinical judgments, and management of ethical issues.

The plastic surgery nurse maintains the plastic surgery standards of practice and standards of professional performance in each type of practice environment to help ensure the safety, quality of care, and the highest level of health maintenance or health restoration for the consumer undergoing plastic surgery. The plastic surgery nurse's attitude and performance reflect compassion and understanding of a consumer's self-respect, cultural beliefs, sovereignty, and rights to self-determination and privacy. Plastic surgery nurses implement the principles of autonomy, nonmaleficence, beneficence, and justice when interacting with consumers requiring or desiring plastic surgery interventions. Plastic surgery nurses are aware of the many ethical considerations associated with the public's perception of plastic surgery, which include misleading advertising, issues affecting the aging population, insurance reimbursement, and other matters. Public awareness of these issues is the key to proper acknowledgment of the physical and emotional health concerns and risks of plastic surgery.

Misleading Advertising

Advertisements for plastic surgery are found in print, broadcast media, and the Internet. Many plastic or cosmetic surgery advertisements do not disclose risks, recovery time, contraindications, physician credentials, type of board certification, or type of surgical facility. Plastic surgery nurses encourage consumers who are interested in plastic surgery to inquire about the physician, the surgical environment, and the procedure in detail, in order to make an informed decision. Although the American Board of Plastic Surgery (www.abps .org) recognizes the role of legitimate advertising in the changing medical scene, it does not approve of plastic surgery advertising that is false or misleading and minimizes the magnitude and possible risks of surgery, or which solicits healthcare consumers for operations that they might not otherwise consider. Public awareness of plastic surgery advertising, in general, is a focus of plastic surgery nursing education in community campaigns.

The Aging Population

The quest for a more youthful appearance to complement longevity is spreading among the aging population in our society. Aging adults are considered vulnerable because of age-related physical and cognitive changes that make them more susceptible to health risks during and after surgery. According to the ASPS statistical chart for age distribution (2009), consumers aged 55 and older underwent 3.1 million total cosmetic procedures, of which 344,000 were surgical and 2.8 million were minimally invasive (www.asps.org). Cosmetic minimally invasive procedures, in general, increased 99% from 2000 to 2009. Plastic surgery nurses must be aware of the specialized needs of the aging population, as well as the ethical considerations associated with their aesthetic surgery requests.

Insurance Reimbursements

Reimbursement for plastic surgery procedures is best facilitated by educating insurance providers as to the differences between cosmetic and reconstructive surgery. Cosmetic surgery seeks to improve the patient's features on a purely aesthetic level, in the absence of any actual deformity or trauma. For this reason, insurance companies normally do not cover cosmetic surgery. In contrast, the purpose of reconstructive surgery is to correct any physical feature that is grossly deformed or abnormal by accepted standards—either as the result of a birth defect, illness, or trauma. Often, reconstructive surgery not only addresses the deformed appearance, but also seeks to correct or improve some deficiency or abnormality in function as well. A plastic surgery nurse in a plastic surgery practice environment is in a unique position to act as a consumer advocate or a change agent to help secure insurance reimbursements for those undergoing such reconstructive procedures.

Summary of the Scope of Plastic Surgery Nursing Practice

Plastic surgery nursing specializes in the protection, maintenance, safety, and optimization of health and human bodily restoration and repair before, during, and after plastic surgery cosmetic, reconstructive, and nonsurgical aesthetic procedures, regardless of the practice environment. The plastic surgery nurse collaborates, consults, and serves as a liaison and advocate for individuals, families, communities, and populations. With the dynamic and ever-changing healthcare practice environment, the plastic surgery nurse is constantly seeking to utilize the best available evidence to guide practice and promote optimal consumer outcomes for the whole person.

Standards of Plastic Surgery Nursing Practice

Standards of Practice for Plastic Surgery Nursing

Standard 1. Assessment

The plastic surgery registered nurse collects comprehensive data pertinent to the healthcare consumer's health and/or situation.

COMPETENCIES

The plastic surgery nurse:

- Collects comprehensive data, including but not limited to physical, functional, psychosocial, emotional, cognitive, sexual, cultural, age-related, environmental, spiritual/transpersonal, and economic assessments, in a systematic and ongoing process while honoring the uniqueness of the person.

- Elicits the healthcare consumer's values, preferences, expressed needs, expectations, and knowledge of the healthcare situation.

- Identifies barriers to effective communication and makes appropriate adaptations.

- Includes the healthcare consumer, family, significant others, and appropriate healthcare providers in the holistic data collection process.

- Recognizes the impact of personal attitudes, values, and beliefs.

- Prioritizes data collection.

- Uses appropriate evidence-based assessment techniques, analytical models and instruments, and problem-solving tools in collecting pertinent data according to the plastic surgery healthcare consumer's immediate health condition, situation, or anticipated needs.

- Synthesizes available data, information, and knowledge relevant to the situation to identify patterns and variances.

- Documents relevant data in a retrievable format.

- Applies ethical, legal, and privacy guidelines and policies to the collection, maintenance, use, and dissemination of data and information.

- Recognizes the healthcare consumer as the authority on her or his own health by honoring the consumer's care preferences.

- Assesses family dynamics and impact on healthcare consumer health and wellness.

ADDITIONAL COMPETENCIES FOR THE ADVANCED PRACTICE REGISTERED NURSE IN PLASTIC SURGERY

The advanced practice registered nurse in plastic surgery:

- Conducts in-depth and comprehensive assessments based on a synthesis of individual and family health.

- Bases assessments on advanced knowledge in the field of plastic surgery.

- Initiates and interprets diagnostic tests and procedures relevant to the current status of the plastic surgery healthcare consumer.

- Assesses the effect of interactions among individuals, family, community, and social systems on health and illness.

Standard 2. Diagnosis

The plastic surgery registered nurse analyzes the assessment data to determine the diagnoses or issues.

COMPETENCIES

The plastic surgery registered nurse:

- Derives the diagnosis and issues from the assessment data obtained during interview, consultation, physical examination, diagnostic test, or diagnostic procedures.

- Identifies actual or potential risks to the healthcare consumer's health and safety, as well as barriers to health, which may include but are not limited to interpersonal, systematic, or environmental circumstances.

- Uses standardized classification systems and clinical decision support tools, when available, in identifying diagnoses.

- Bases the diagnosis on actual or potential responses to alterations in health.

- Validates the diagnoses or issues with the plastic surgery healthcare consumer, significant others, and other appropriate healthcare providers when possible.

- Documents diagnoses or issues in a manner that facilitates determination of the expected outcomes and plan.

ADDITIONAL COMPETENCIES FOR THE ADVANCED PRACTICE REGISTERED NURSE IN PLASTIC SURGERY

The advanced practice registered nurse in plastic surgery:

- Systematically compares and contrasts clinical findings of the plastic surgery patient with normal and abnormal variations and developmental events when formulating a differential diagnosis.

- Utilizes complex data and information obtained during the interview, consultation, examination, and diagnostic procedures, and initiates further appropriate diagnostic tests to complete the identification of diagnoses.

- Assists staff in building and sustaining competency in the diagnostic process.

Standard 3. Outcomes Identification

The plastic surgery registered nurse identifies expected outcomes for a plan individualized to the healthcare consumer or the situation.

COMPETENCIES

The plastic surgery registered nurse:

- Involves the healthcare consumer, family, healthcare providers, and others in formulating expected outcomes when possible and appropriate.

- Derives culturally appropriate expected outcomes from the diagnoses.

- Considers associated risks, benefits, costs, current scientific evidence, expected trajectory of the condition, and clinical expertise when formulating expected outcomes.

- Defines expected outcomes in terms of the healthcare consumer's culture, values, and ethical considerations.

- Includes a time estimate for the attainment of expected outcomes.

- Develops expected outcomes that facilitate continuity of care.

- Modifies expected outcomes based on changes in the status of the healthcare consumer or evaluation of the situation.

- Documents expected outcomes as measurable goals.

ADDITIONAL COMPETENCIES FOR THE ADVANCED PRACTICE REGISTERED NURSE IN PLASTIC SURGERY

The advanced practice registered nurse in plastic surgery:

- Identifies expected outcomes that incorporate scientific evidence and are achievable through implementation of evidence-based practices.

- Identifies expected outcomes that incorporate cost and clinical effectiveness, healthcare consumer satisfaction, and continuity and consistency among providers.

- Differentiates outcomes that require care process interventions from those that require system-level interventions.

Standard 4. Planning

The plastic surgery registered nurse develops a plan that prescribes strategies and alternatives to attain expected outcomes.

COMPETENCIES

The plastic surgery registered nurse:

- Develops an individualized plan in partnership with the healthcare consumer, family, and others while considering the healthcare consumer's characteristics or situation, including but not limited to values, beliefs, spiritual and health practices, preferences, choices, developmental level, coping style, culture and environment, and available technology.

- Establishes the plan priorities with the healthcare consumer, family, and others as appropriate.

- Includes strategies in the plan that address each of the identified diagnoses or issues. These may include, but are not limited to, strategies for:

  - Promotion and restoration of health

  - Prevention of illness, injury, and disease

  - Alleviation of suffering

  - Supportive care for those who are dying

- Includes strategies for health and wholeness across the lifespan.

- Provides for continuity in the plan.

- Incorporates an implementation pathway or timeline in the plan.

- Utilizes the plan to provide direction to other members of the healthcare team.

- Explores practice settings and safe space and time for the plastic surgery registered nurse and the healthcare consumer to explore suggested, potential, and alternative options.

- Defines a plan that reflects current statutes, rules, regulations, standards, and policies.

- Modifies the plan according to ongoing assessment of the healthcare consumer's response and other outcome indicators.

- Integrates current scientific evidence, trends, and research in the planning process.

- Considers the economic impact of the plan on the plastic surgery patient, family, caregivers, and other affected parties.

- Documents the plan in a manner that uses standardized language or recognized terminology.

ADDITIONAL COMPETENCIES FOR THE ADVANCED PRACTICE REGISTERED NURSE IN PLASTIC SURGERY

The advanced practice registered nurse in plastic surgery:

- Identifies assessment and diagnostic strategies and therapeutic interventions in the plan that reflect current evidence, including data, research, literature, and expert clinical knowledge.

- Selects or designs strategies to meet the multifaceted needs of complex plastic surgery healthcare consumers.

- Includes a synthesis of the healthcare consumer's values and beliefs regarding nursing and medical therapies within the plan.

- Actively participates in the development and continuous improvement of systems that support the planning process.

- Leads the design and development of interprofessional processes to address the identified diagnosis or issue.

Standard 5. Implementation

The plastic surgery registered nurse implements the identified plan.

COMPETENCIES

The plastic surgery registered nurse:

- Partners with the person, family, significant others, and caregivers as appropriate to implement the plan in a safe, realistic, and timely manner.

- Demonstrates caring behaviors toward healthcare consumers, significant others, and groups of people receiving care.

- Utilizes technology to measure, record, and retrieve healthcare consumer data, implement the nursing process, and enhance plastic surgery nursing practice.

- Utilizes evidence-based interventions and treatments specific to the diagnosis or problem of the plastic surgery healthcare consumer.

- Provides holistic care that addresses the needs of diverse populations across the lifespan.

- Advocates for health care that is sensitive to the needs of healthcare consumers, with particular emphasis on the needs of diverse populations.

- Applies appropriate knowledge of major health problems and cultural diversity in implementing the plan of care.

- Applies available healthcare technologies to maximize access and optimize outcomes for healthcare consumers.

- Utilizes community resources and systems to implement the plan.

- Collaborates with healthcare providers from diverse backgrounds to implement and integrate the plan.

- Accommodates different styles of communication used by healthcare consumers, families, and healthcare providers.

- Integrates traditional and complementary healthcare practices as appropriate.

- Implements the plan in a timely manner in accordance with healthcare consumer safety goals.

- Promotes the healthcare consumer's capacity for the optimal level of participation and problem-solving.

- Documents implementation and any modifications, including changes or omissions, of the identified plan.

ADDITIONAL COMPETENCIES FOR THE ADVANCED PRACTICE REGISTERED NURSE IN PLASTIC SURGERY

The advanced practice registered nurse in plastic surgery:

- Facilitates utilization of systems, organizations, and community resources to implement the plan for the plastic surgery healthcare consumer.

- Supports collaboration with nursing and other colleagues to implement the plan.

- Incorporates new knowledge and strategies to initiate change in plastic surgery nursing care practices if desired outcomes are not achieved.

- Assumes responsibility for safe and efficient implementation of the plan.

- Uses advanced communication skills to promote relationships between plastic surgery nurses and healthcare consumers, to provide a context for open discussion of the healthcare consumer's experiences, and to improve healthcare consumer outcomes.

- Actively participates in the development and continuous improvement of systems that support implementation of the plan.

Standard 5A. Coordination of Care

The plastic surgery registered nurse coordinates care delivery.

COMPETENCIES

The plastic surgery registered nurse:

- Organizes the components of the plan.

- Manages a healthcare consumer's care so as to maximize independence and quality of life.

- Assists the healthcare consumer in identifying options for alternative care.

- Communicates with the healthcare consumer, family, and system during transitions in care.

- Advocates for the delivery of dignified and humane care by the interprofessional team.

- Documents the coordination of the care.

ADDITIONAL COMPETENCIES FOR THE ADVANCED PRACTICE REGISTERED NURSE IN PLASTIC SURGERY

The advanced practice registered nurse in plastic surgery:

- Provides leadership in the coordination of interprofessional heath care for integrated delivery of plastic surgery healthcare consumer care services.

- Synthesizes data and information to prescribe necessary system and community support measures, including modifications of surroundings.

Standard 5B. Health Teaching and Health Promotion

The plastic surgery registered nurse employs strategies to promote health and a safe environment.

COMPETENCIES

The plastic surgery registered nurse:

- Provides health teaching that addresses such topics as healthy lifestyles, risk-reducing behaviors, developmental needs, activities of daily living, and preventive self-care.

- Uses health promotion and health teaching methods appropriate to the situation and the healthcare consumer's values, beliefs, health practices, developmental level, learning needs, readiness and ability to learn, language preference, spirituality, culture, and socioeconomic status.

- Seeks opportunities for feedback and evaluation of the effectiveness of the strategies used.

- Uses information technologies to communicate health promotion and disease prevention information to the healthcare consumer in a variety of settings.

- Provides healthcare consumers with information about intended effects and potential adverse effects of proposed therapies.

ADDITIONAL COMPETENCIES FOR THE ADVANCED PRACTICE REGISTERED NURSE IN PLASTIC SURGERY

The advanced practice registered nurse in plastic surgery:

- Synthesizes empirical evidence on risk behaviors, learning theories, behavioral change theories, motivational theories, epidemiology, and other related theories and frameworks when designing health information and programs.

- Conducts personalized health teaching and counseling in accordance with comparative effectiveness research recommendations.

- Designs health information and healthcare consumer education appropriate to the healthcare consumer's developmental level, learning needs, readiness to learn, and cultural values and beliefs.

- Evaluates health information resources, such as the Internet, within the area of plastic surgery nursing practice for accuracy, readability, and comprehensibility, to help healthcare consumers access quality health information.

- Engages consumer alliances and advocacy groups, as appropriate, in health teaching and health promotion activities.

- Provides anticipatory guidance to individuals, families, groups, and communities to promote health and prevent or reduce the risk of health problems.

Standard 5C. Consultation

The advanced practice registered nurse in plastic surgery provides consultation to influence the specified plan, enhance the abilities of others, and effect change.

COMPETENCIES FOR THE ADVANCED PRACTICE REGISTERED NURSE

The advanced practice registered nurse in plastic surgery:

- Synthesizes clinical data, theoretical frameworks, and evidence when providing consultation.

- Facilitates the effectiveness of a consultation by involving the healthcare consumer and other stakeholders in the decision-making process and negotiating role responsibilities.

- Communicates consultation recommendations.

Standard 5D. Prescriptive Authority and Treatment

The advanced practice registered nurse in plastic surgery uses prescriptive authority, procedures, referrals, treatments, and therapies in accordance with state and federal laws and regulations.

COMPETENCIES FOR THE ADVANCED PRACTICE REGISTERED NURSE

The advanced practice registered nurse in plastic surgery:

- Prescribes evidence-based treatments, therapies, and procedures considering the healthcare consumer's comprehensive healthcare needs.

- Prescribes pharmacological agents based on current knowledge of pharmacology and physiology.

- Prescribes specific pharmacological agents and/or treatments according to clinical indicators, the healthcare consumer's status and needs, and the results of diagnostic and laboratory tests.

- Evaluates therapeutic and potential adverse effects of pharmacological and nonpharmacological treatments.

- Provides healthcare consumers with information about intended effects and potential adverse effects of proposed prescriptive therapies.

- Provides information about costs and alternative treatments and procedures, as appropriate.

- Evaluates and incorporates complementary and alternative therapy into education and practice.

Standard 6. Evaluation

The plastic surgery nurse evaluates progress toward attainment of outcomes.

COMPETENCIES

The plastic surgery registered nurse:

- Conducts a systematic, ongoing, and criterion-based evaluation of the outcomes in relation to the structures and processes prescribed by the plan of care and the indicated timeline.

- Collaborates with the healthcare consumer and others involved in the care or situation in the evaluation process.

- Evaluates, in partnership with the healthcare consumer, the effectiveness of the planned strategies in relation to the healthcare consumer's responses and attainment of the expected outcomes.

- Documents the results of the evaluation.

- Uses ongoing assessment data to revise the diagnoses, outcomes, plan of care, and implementation as needed.

- Disseminates the results to the healthcare consumer, family, and others involved, in accordance with federal and state regulations.

- Participates in assessing and assuring the responsible and appropriate use of interventions in order to minimize unwarranted or unwanted treatment and healthcare consumer suffering.

ADDITIONAL COMPETENCIES FOR THE ADVANCED PRACTICE REGISTERED NURSE IN PLASTIC SURGERY

The advanced practice registered nurse in plastic surgery:

- Evaluates the accuracy of the diagnosis and effectiveness of the interventions and other variables in relation to the healthcare consumer's attainment of expected outcomes.

- Adapts the plan of care for the trajectory of treatment according to the evaluation of response.

■ Synthesizes the results of the evaluation to determine the effect of the plan on healthcare consumers, families, groups, communities, and institutions.

■ Uses the results of the evaluation to make or recommend process or structural changes, including policy, procedure, or protocol revision, as appropriate.

Standards of Professional Performance for Plastic Surgery Nursing

Standard 7. Ethics

The plastic surgery registered nurse practices ethically.

COMPETENCIES

The plastic surgery registered nurse:

- Uses *Code of Ethics for Nurses with Interpretive Statements* (ANA, 2001) to guide practice.

- Delivers care in a manner that preserves and protects healthcare consumer autonomy, dignity, rights, values, and beliefs.

- Recognizes the centrality of the healthcare consumer and family as core members of the healthcare team.

- Upholds healthcare consumer confidentiality within legal and regulatory parameters.

- Assists healthcare consumers in self-determination and informed decision-making.

- Maintains a therapeutic and professional healthcare consumer–nurse relationship within appropriate professional role boundaries.

- Contributes to resolving ethical issues involving healthcare consumers, colleagues, community groups, systems, and other stakeholders.

- Takes appropriate action regarding instances of illegal, unethical, or inappropriate behavior that could endanger or jeopardize the best interests of the healthcare consumer or situation.

- Speaks up as appropriate to question healthcare practice, when necessary for safety and quality improvement.

- Advocates for equitable healthcare consumer care.

ADDITIONAL COMPETENCIES FOR THE ADVANCED PRACTICE REGISTERED NURSE IN PLASTIC SURGERY

The advanced practice registered nurse in plastic surgery:

- Provides information on the risks, benefits, and outcomes of the healthcare consumer regimens to allow informed decision-making by the healthcare consumer, including informed consent and informed refusal.

- Participates in interprofessional teams that address ethical risks, benefits, and outcomes.

Standard 8. Education

The plastic surgery registered nurse attains knowledge and competence that reflect current plastic surgery nursing practice.

COMPETENCIES

The plastic surgery registered nurse:

- Participates in ongoing educational activities related to appropriate knowledge bases and professional issues.

- Demonstrates a commitment to lifelong learning through self-reflection and inquiry to address learning and personal growth needs.

- Seeks experiences that reflect current plastic surgery nursing practice, to maintain knowledge, skills, abilities, and judgment in clinical practice or role performance.

- Acquires knowledge and skills appropriate to the role, population, specialty, setting, or situation.

- Seeks formal and independent learning experiences to develop and maintain clinical and professional skills and knowledge.

- Identifies learning needs based on nursing knowledge, the various roles the plastic surgery registered nurse may assume, and the changing needs of the population.

- Participates in formal or informal consultations to address issues in plastic surgery nursing practice as an application of education and a knowledge base.

- Shares educational findings, experiences, and ideas with peers.

- Contributes to a work environment conducive to the education of healthcare professionals.

- Maintains professional records that provide evidence of competence and lifelong learning.

ADDITIONAL COMPETENCIES FOR THE ADVANCED PRACTICE REGISTERED NURSE IN PLASTIC SURGERY

The advanced practice registered nurse in plastic surgery:

- Uses current healthcare research findings and other evidence to expand clinical knowledge, skills, abilities, and judgment to enhance role performance, and to increase knowledge of professional issues.

Standard 9. Evidence-Based Practice and Research

The plastic surgery registered nurse integrates evidence and research findings into practice.

COMPETENCIES

The plastic surgery registered nurse:

- Utilizes current evidence-based nursing knowledge, including research findings, to guide practice.

- Incorporates evidence when initiating changes in plastic surgery nursing practice.

- Participates, as appropriate to education level and position, in the formulation of evidence-based practice through research.

- Shares personal and third-party research findings with colleagues and peers.

ADDITIONAL COMPETENCIES FOR THE ADVANCED PRACTICE REGISTERED NURSE IN PLASTIC SURGERY

The advanced practice registered nurse in plastic surgery:

- Contributes to plastic surgery nursing knowledge by conducting or synthesizing research and other evidence that discovers, examines, and evaluates current practice, knowledge, theories, criteria, and creative approaches to improve healthcare outcomes.

- Promotes a climate of research and clinical inquiry.

- Disseminates research findings through activities such as presentations, publications, consultation, and journal clubs.

Standard 10. Quality of Practice

The plastic surgery registered nurse contributes to quality nursing practice.

COMPETENCIES

The plastic surgery registered nurse:

- Demonstrates quality by documenting the application of the nursing process in a responsible, accountable, and ethical manner,

- Uses creativity and innovation to enhance plastic surgery nursing care.

- Participates in quality improvement activities, such as but not limited to:

  - Identifying aspects of practice important for quality monitoring

  - Using indicators to monitor quality, safety, and effectiveness of plastic surgery nursing practice

  - Collecting data to monitor quality and effectiveness of plastic surgery nursing practice

  - Analyzing quality data to identify opportunities for improving plastic surgery nursing practice

  - Formulating recommendations to improve plastic surgery nursing practice or outcomes

  - Implementing activities to enhance the quality of plastic surgery nursing practice

  - Developing, implementing, and/or evaluating policies, procedures, and guidelines to improve the quality of practice

  - Participating in and/or leading interprofessional teams to evaluate clinical care or health services

  - Participating in and/or leading efforts to minimize costs and unnecessary duplication

  - Identifying problems that occur in day-to-day work routines, in order to correct process inefficiencies

  - Analyzing factors related to quality, safety, and effectiveness

- Analyzing organizational systems for barriers to quality healthcare consumer outcomes

- Implementing processes to remove or weaken barriers within organizational systems

- Obtains and maintains professional certification in plastic surgery nursing.

ADDITIONAL COMPETENCIES FOR THE ADVANCED PRACTICE REGISTERED NURSE IN PLASTIC SURGERY

The advanced practice registered nurse in plastic surgery:

- Provides leadership in design and implementation of quality improvements.

- Designs innovations to effect change in practice and improve health outcomes.

- Evaluates the practice environment and quality of nursing care rendered in relation to existing evidence.

- Identifies opportunities for the generation and use of research and evidence.

- Obtains and maintains professional certification.

- Uses the results of quality improvement to initiate changes in plastic surgery nursing practice and the healthcare delivery system.

Standard 11. Communication

The plastic surgery registered nurse communicates effectively in a variety of formats in all areas of practice.

COMPETENCIES
The plastic surgery registered nurse:

- Assesses communication format preferences of healthcare consumers, families, and colleagues.

- Assesses her or his own communication skills in encounters with healthcare consumers, families, and colleagues.

- Seeks continuous improvement of communication and conflict resolution skills.

- Conveys information to healthcare consumers, families, the interprofessional team, and others in communication formats that promote accuracy.

- Questions the rationale supporting care processes and decisions when they do not appear to be in the best interest of the plastic surgery healthcare consumer.

- Discloses observations or concerns related to hazards and errors in care or the practice environment to the appropriate level.

- Maintains communication with other providers to minimize risks associated with transfers and transition in care delivery.

- Contributes her or his own professional perspective in discussions with the interprofessional team.

Standard 12. Leadership

The plastic surgery nurse demonstrates leadership in the professional practice setting and in the profession.

COMPETENCIES

The plastic surgery registered nurse:

- Oversees the nursing care given by others while retaining accountability for the quality of care given to the healthcare consumer.

- Abides by the vision, the associated goals, and the plan to implement and measure progress of an individual healthcare consumer or progress within the context of the healthcare organization.

- Demonstrates a commitment to continuous, lifelong learning and education for self and others.

- Mentors colleagues for advancement of plastic surgery nursing practice, the profession, and quality health care.

- Treats colleagues with respect, trust, and dignity.

- Develops communication and conflict resolution skills.

- Participates in professional organizations, including the American Society of Plastic Surgical Nurses.

- Communicates effectively with the healthcare consumer and colleagues.

- Seeks ways to advance plastic surgery nursing autonomy and accountability.

- Participates in efforts to influence healthcare policy involving healthcare consumers and plastic surgery nursing.

ADDITIONAL COMPETENCIES FOR THE ADVANCED PRACTICE REGISTERED NURSE IN PLASTIC SURGERY

The advanced practice registered nurse in plastic surgery:

- Influences decision-making bodies to improve the professional practice environment and healthcare consumer outcomes.

- Provides direction to enhance the effectiveness of the interprofessional team.

■ Promotes advanced practice in plastic surgery nursing and role development by interpreting its role for the healthcare consumer, families, and others.

■ Models expert practice to interprofessional team members and healthcare consumers.

■ Mentors colleagues in the acquisition of clinical knowledge, skills, abilities, and judgment.

Standard 13. Collaboration

The plastic surgery registered nurse collaborates with the healthcare consumer, family, and others in the conduct of plastic surgery nursing practice.

COMPETENCIES

The plastic surgery registered nurse:

- Partners with others to effect change and produce positive outcomes through sharing of knowledge of the healthcare consumer and/or situation.

- Communicates with the healthcare consumer, family, and healthcare providers regarding healthcare consumer care and the plastic surgery registered nurse's role in the provision of that care.

- Promotes conflict management and engagement.

- Participates in building consensus or resolving conflict in the context of patient care.

- Applies group process and negotiation techniques with healthcare consumers and colleagues.

- Adheres to standards and applicable codes of conduct that govern behavior among peers and colleagues, so as to create a work environment that promotes cooperation, respect, and trust.

- Cooperates in creating a documented plan focused on outcomes and decisions related to care and delivery of services that indicates communication with healthcare consumers, families, and others.

- Engages in teamwork and team-building processes.

ADDITIONAL COMPETENCIES FOR THE ADVANCED PRACTICE REGISTERED NURSE IN PLASTIC SURGERY

The advanced practice registered nurse in plastic surgery:

- Partners with other disciplines to enhance healthcare consumer outcomes through interprofessional activities, such as education, consultation, management, technological development, or research opportunities.

- Invites the contribution of the healthcare consumer, family, and team members in order to achieve optimal outcomes.

- Leads in establishing, improving, and sustaining collaborative relationships to achieve safe, quality healthcare consumer care.

- Documents plan-of-care communications, rationales for plan-of-care changes, and collaborative discussions to improve healthcare consumer outcomes.

Standard 14. Professional Practice Evaluation

The plastic surgery registered nurse evaluates her or his own nursing practice in relation to professional practice standards and guidelines, relevant statutes, rules, and regulations.

COMPETENCIES

The plastic surgery registered nurse:

- Provides age-appropriate and developmentally appropriate care in a culturally and ethnically sensitive manner.

- Engages in self-evaluation of practice on a regular basis, identifying areas of strength as well as areas in which professional growth would be beneficial.

- Obtains informal feedback regarding her or his own practice from healthcare consumers, peers, professional colleagues, and others.

- Participates in peer review as appropriate.

- Takes action to achieve goals identified during the evaluation process.

- Provides the evidence for practice decisions and actions as part of the informal and formal evaluation processes.

- Interacts with peers and colleagues to enhance her or his own professional nursing practice or role performance.

- Provides peers with formal or informal constructive feedback regarding their practice and role performance.

ADDITIONAL COMPETENCIES FOR THE ADVANCED PRACTICE REGISTERED NURSE IN PLASTIC SURGERY

The advanced practice registered nurse in plastic surgery:

- Engages in a formal process of seeking feedback regarding her or his own practice from healthcare consumers, peers, professional colleagues, and others.

Standard 15. Resource Utilization

The plastic surgery registered nurse utilizes appropriate resources to plan and provide nursing services that are safe, effective, and financially responsible.

COMPETENCIES
The plastic surgery registered nurse:

- Assesses individual healthcare consumer care needs and resources available to achieve desired outcomes.

- Identifies healthcare consumer care needs, potential for harm, complexity of the task, and desired outcome when considering resource allocation.

- Delegates elements of care to appropriate healthcare workers in accordance with any applicable legal or policy parameters or principles.

- Identifies the evidence when evaluating resources.

- Advocates for resources, including technology, that enhance plastic surgery nursing practice.

- Modifies practice when necessary to promote positive interaction between healthcare consumers, care providers, and technology.

- Assists the healthcare consumer and family in identifying and securing appropriate services to address needs across the healthcare continuum.

- Assists the healthcare consumer and family in factoring costs, risks, and benefits in decisions about treatment and care.

ADDITIONAL COMPETENCIES FOR THE ADVANCED PRACTICE REGISTERED NURSE IN PLASTIC SURGERY
The advanced practice registered nurse in plastic surgery:

- Utilizes organizational and community resources to formulate interprofessional plans of care.

- Formulates innovative solutions for healthcare consumer care problems that utilize resources effectively and maintain quality.

- Designs evaluation strategies to demonstrate cost effectiveness, cost benefit, and efficiency factors associated with plastic surgery nursing practice.

Standard 16. Environmental Health

The plastic surgery registered nurse practices in an environmentally safe and healthy manner.

COMPETENCIES

The plastic surgery registered nurse:

- Attains knowledge of environmental health concepts, such as implementation of environmental health strategies.

- Promotes a practice environment that reduces environmental health risks for workers and healthcare consumers.

- Assesses the practice environment for factors that threaten health, such as sound, odor, noise, and light.

- Advocates for the judicious and appropriate use of products in health care.

- Communicates environmental health risks and exposure reduction strategies to healthcare consumers, families, colleagues, and communities.

- Utilizes scientific evidence to determine if a product or treatment is an environmental threat.

- Participates in strategies to promote healthy communities.

ADDITIONAL COMPETENCIES FOR THE ADVANCED PRACTICE REGISTERED NURSE IN PLASTIC SURGERY

The advanced practice registered nurse in plastic surgery:

- Creates partnerships that promote sustainable environmental health policies and conditions.

- Analyzes the impact of social, political, and economic influences on the environment and human health exposures.

- Critically evaluates the manner in which environmental health issues are presented by the popular media.

- Advocates for implementation of environmental principles for plastic surgery nursing practice.

- Supports nurses in advocating for and implementing environmental principles in plastic surgery nursing practice.

Glossary

Competency. An expected and measurable level of nursing performance that integrates knowledge, skills, abilities, and judgment, based on established scientific knowledge and expectations for nursing practice.

Environment. The surrounding context, milieu, conditions, or atmosphere in which a plastic surgery nurse practices.

Evidence-based practice. A scholarly and systematic problem-solving paradigm that results in the delivery of high-quality health care.

Healthcare team. A set of individuals with special expertise who provide healthcare services or assistance to patients. They may include nurses, physicians, psychologists, social workers, nutritionists/dieticians, and various therapists. Healthcare providers also may include service organizations and vendors. A team is comprised of a number of persons associated together in work or activity.

Holism (holistic). A view of everything in terms of patterns and processes that combine to form a whole, instead of seeing things as fragments, pieces, or parts. Holistic nursing embraces nursing practice, which has healing the whole person as its goal. Holism involves understanding the individual as an integrated whole interacting with and being acted upon by both internal and external environments.

Interprofessional. Reliant on the overlapping knowledge, skills, and abilities of each professional team member. Interprofessionalism can drive synergistic effects by which outcomes are enhanced and become more comprehensive than a simple aggregation of the individual efforts of the team members.

Plastic surgery nursing. An area of nursing that specializes in the protection, maintenance, safety, and optimization of human bodily repair, restoration, and health before, during, and after plastic surgery procedures. This is accomplished through the nursing process, nursing diagnosis, and treatment of human response.

Role. A function; specifically, the characteristic and expected social behavior of an individual in relationship to a group.

Standards. Authoritative statements defined and promoted by a profession by which the quality of practice, service, or education can be evaluated.

References

American Board of Medical Specialties (ABMS). (2000). *Member boards and associate members.* Available at http://www.abms.org/member.asp

American Board of Plastic Surgery. (2011). *About ABPS.* Available at http://www.abplsurg.org/about_abps.html#Description%20of%20Plastic%20Surgery

American Nurses Association (ANA). (2001). *Code of Ethics for Nurses with interpretive statements.* Washington, DC: ANA.

American Nurses Association (ANA). (2010a). *Nursing: Scope and standards of practice, 2nd ed.* Silver Spring, MD: Nursesbooks.org.

American Nurses Association (ANA). (2010b). *Nursing's social policy statement: The essence of the profession.* Silver Spring, MD: Nursesbooks.org

Association of periOperative Registered Nurses (AORN). (2011). *Standards and recommended practices.* Available at www.aorn.org

American Society of Plastic Surgeons. (2009). *Plastic surgery procedural statistics.* Available at http://www.plasticsurgery.org/News-and-Resources/Statistics.html

American Society of Plastic Surgical Nurses (ASPSN). (2010). *About ASPSN.* Available at http://www.aspsn.org/ABOUT/objectives.html

Appendix A.

Plastic Surgery Nursing: Scope and Standards of Practice (2005)

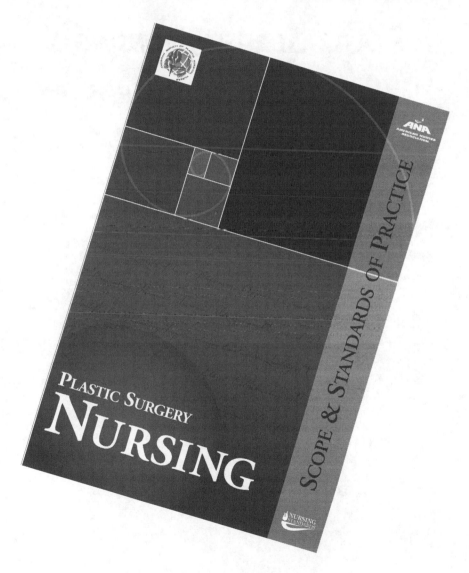

The content in this appendix is not current and is of historical significance only.

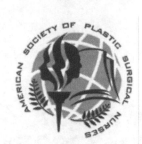

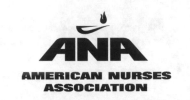

AMERICAN NURSES ASSOCIATION

PLASTIC SURGERY NURSING:

SCOPE AND STANDARDS

OF PRACTICE

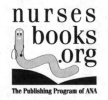

The Publishing Program of ANA

AMERICAN NURSES ASSOCIATION
Silver Spring, MD
2005

The content in this appendix is not current and is of historical significance only.

Contents

The content in this appendix is not current and is of historical significance only.

The content in this appendix is not current and is of historical significance only.

ACKNOWLEDGMENTS

Sharon Fritzsche, RN, MSN, APRN,BC
Judy Akin, RN, MSN, PHN

Special thanks to the Clinical Practice Committee Chairman Sharon D. Fritzsche MSN, RN, APRN,BC, and committee member Judy Akin, RN, MSN, PHN of the ASPSN for their invaluable insight and commitment to having the ASPSN be recognized as a specialty organization by the ANA. The ASPSN would also like to give thanks to Carol J. Bickford, PhD, RN, BC, Senior Policy Fellow, Department of Nursing Practice and Economics, for her guidance and reference in the development of the Scope of Practice Statement and revision of the Standards of Practice and Professional Performance for the ASPSN.

ANA Staff

Carol J. Bickford, PhD, RN,BC – Content Editor
Yvonne Humes, MSA
Winifred Carson, JD

The content in this appendix is not current and is of historical significance only.

SCOPE OF PLASTIC SURGERY NURSING PRACTICE

Definition of Plastic Surgery Nursing

Plastic surgery nursing specializes in the protection, maintenance, safety, and optimization of human bodily repair, restoration, and health before, during, and after plastic surgery procedures. This is accomplished through the nursing process, nursing diagnosis, and treatment of human response. Commitment to the nursing profession is reflected in service and advocacy for individuals, families, communities, and populations through to care, education, and ethics of plastic surgery issues and procedures.

Foundation of Plastic Surgery Nursing Practice

The specialty of plastic surgery has long pioneered surgical techniques and treatment strategies for human body and facial repair, reconstruction and replacement in cases of congenital diseases, traumatic injuries, and cancer reconstruction. Plastic surgery encompasses the skin, breast, trunk, craniomaxillofacial structures, musculoskeletal system, extremities, and external genitalia. Complex wounds, replantation, grafts, flaps, free tissue transfer, and use of implantable materials are also functions of plastic surgery surgical residencies. In addition, plastic surgery has extended surgical reconstruction to aid in the correction or enhancement of aesthetic surgical issues (American Board of Plastic Surgery 2003). Plastic surgery interventions encompass all ages, from the neonatal patient to the advanced geriatric patient. This requires specialized knowledge and treatment to ensure optimal patient outcomes. Plastic surgery is the only specialty recognized and supported by the American Board of Medical Specialties (ABMS 2000) that provides plastic, reconstructive, and aesthetic surgical procedures through board certification for plastic surgery.

Unfortunately, because of extensive media coverage of plastic surgery and increasing demands for aesthetic plastic surgery, procedures are being performed by other medical specialties without properly recognized or regulated board certifications or surgical residencies. The lack of regulation, specialized knowledge, and skill levels exposes individuals,

The content in this appendix is not current and is of historical significance only.

families, communities, and populations to unnecessary health and safety risks. Plastic surgery nurses are aware of the health risks associated with plastic surgery procedures. Plastic surgery nurses complement the plastic surgery specialty by a mutual focus on patient safety, health maintenance, and ultimate patient satisfaction and outcomes.

Plastic surgery nursing practice and standards reflect the nursing process, the nursing standards of both the American Nurses Association (ANA 1995, 2000, 2004), and the Association of periOperative Registered Nurses (AORN) standards of perioperative practice, and AORN standards of nursing practice (AORN 2001). Plastic surgery nursing requires specialized knowledge and skill levels for both the reconstructive and aesthetic aspects of surgical interventions during the consultation, preoperative, operative, and postoperative stages of the plastic surgery procedure process. Through the implementation and maintenance of specialized plastic surgery nursing standards of care and practice, individuals seeking or requiring plastic surgery intervention will be provided with education, knowledge, and care to ensure optimal surgical safety, protection, and outcomes.

Development of Plastic Surgery Nursing Practice

Plastic surgery nursing opportunities continue to expand as the demand for plastic surgery procedures and treatments grows, primarily in the United States. According to the American Society of Plastic Surgeons (ASPS 2004), over 15 million plastic surgery procedures and treatments were performed in 2003, compared to approximately 1.5 million in 1992. The need for awareness and knowledge of safety, ethical, and procedural issues will increase as plastic surgery becomes more common in a wide range of surgical environments.

As plastic surgery procedures increase, plastic surgery nursing will intersect with other specialties and bodies of knowledge. These specialties include, but are not limited to, neonatal, pediatrics, adults, geriatrics, general surgery, neurosurgery, advanced wound management, dermatology, burns, cancer, and trauma. Because of the physical and psychological complexities involved in caring for the plastic surgery patient, plastic surgery nursing integrates a holistic approach in the plan of care for the plastic surgery patient. Plastic surgery nursing skills and knowledge require a strong foundation in surgical principles, advanced wound care, bioethics, psychology, and critical thinking.

The content in this appendix is not current and is of historical significance only.

In response to the specialized needs of plastic surgery patients and the required nursing interventions, 100 surgical nurses convened in 1975 to establish the non-profit American Society of Plastic and Reconstructive Surgical Nurses (ASPRSN): the name was later changed to American Society of Plastic Surgical Nurses or ASPSN. These charter members sought to establish a specialized identity and share the knowledge needed to practice successfully. The mission and philosophy of the ASPSN were founded on principles of improving the quality of nursing care for the patient undergoing plastic or reconstructive surgery. The organization is committed to promoting high standards of nursing care and practice through shared knowledge, scientific inquiry, and continuing education, while supporting and encouraging collaborative interaction with clinical practice, administration, research, and academics (ASPSN 2002). The chronology of the development of plastic surgery nursing is summarized on page 4.

Today the ASPSN has over 1,700 active members working in various nursing environments: surgical facilities, home care, nursing research, outpatient care, hospitals, universities, private practice, and others. Members cover a wide range of educational levels, including associate degree, bachelor's degree, master's degree, advanced practice nurses, nurse first-assistants, and nurse educators. ASPSN serves its members through a national structure of four regions and a network of local chapters in the United States and Canada (ASPSN 2002). Through the development of unique plastic surgery knowledge, the plastic surgery nurse can properly respond to and communicate with a multidisciplinary team assigned to any plastic surgery patient.

As the field of plastic surgery evolves and incorporates other medical specialties, the climate for plastic surgery nursing requires continual review of related trends, products, and procedures. According to the current statistical data found on the ASPS and ASPSN web sites, new developments in plastic surgery include both surgical and non-surgical procedures and treatments. Between 1992 and 2002, tumor removal increased 35%, breast reconstruction 147%, scar revision 20%, and animal bite repair 35%. Aesthetic procedures showed an enormous increase between 1992 and 2002, with breast augmentation up 593%, breast lifts 575%, eyelid surgery 91%, facelifts 84%, forehead lifts 176%, buttock lifts 377%, and abdominoplasty 392%. Non-surgical treatments such as collagen injection increased by 139% in the same period. Some of the newest treatments increased dramatically in 2001 and 2002. These

The content in this appendix is not current and is of historical significance only.

include Botox® injections—up 83%—and microdermabrasion—up 39% (ASPS 2004).

Development of Plastic Surgery Nursing

1975   The American Society of Plastic and Reconstructive Surgical Nurses (ASPRSN) holds its first national meeting in Toronto, Canada. Sherill Lee Schultz is the first president and founder.

1976   Thirteen local chapters of ASPRSN are established in the United States and Canada.

1980   ASPRSN creates the *Plastic Surgical Nursing Journal.*

1980   ASPRSN becomes the 22nd member of the National Federation for Specialty Nursing Organizations.

1984   The plastic surgical nursing bibliography is completed.

1989   The first edition of the *Core Curriculum for Plastic and Reconstructive Surgical Nursing* is published in1989 The Plastic Surgical Nursing Certification Board (PSNCB) is established.

1991   The first plastic surgical nursing certification examination (CPSN) is given.

1993   The National Institute of Nursing Research (NINR) is founded and helps move nursing research into the mainstream of research activities.

1995   ASPRSN establishes a Research Committee to assist ASPRSN nurses with research funds and priorities unique to plastic surgical nursing practice.

1996   The second edition of the *Core Curriculum for Plastic and Reconstructive Surgical Nursing* is published.

1998   ASPRSN creates a website: www.aspsn.org

2001   ASPRSN simplifies its name to the American Society of Plastic Surgical Nurses (ASPSN).

2004   Recognition of the specialty and drafting of the ASPSN–ANA specialty standards, *Surgical Nursing: Scope and Standards of Practice*

The content in this appendix is not current and is of historical significance only.

Plastic surgery nurses help to regulate quality of care before, during, and after plastic surgical procedures and treatments to ensure proper health maintenance, safety, and restoration. Plastic surgery nurses determine the specific nursing intervention needed for each individual undergoing a plastic surgical procedure or treatment, in accordance with the nursing process (assessment, diagnosis, outcome identification, planning, implementation, and evaluation). This nursing specialty continues to develop the knowledge base for evidence-based practice through research into plastic surgery procedures, treatments, and issues.

One goal of plastic surgery nursing is to secure the foundation for safety. This is accomplished through stronger regulations, increased education, and awareness among patients, families, communities, and populations seeking or requiring plastic surgery-related interventions.

Educational Preparation and Requirements for Plastic Surgery Nursing

Plastic surgery nursing training embodies *Nursing's Social Policy Statement* (ANA 2003) from novice to expert nursing practice. Advanced education and nursing practice in plastic surgery build on generic practice. Education, experience, and increased familiarity with plastic surgery procedures and outcomes will increase knowledge and skill levels needed to care for the plastic surgery patient.

Due to the complexities of plastic surgery, including psychological and psychosocial factors, plastic surgery nurses require a minimum of two years of basic surgical nursing experience before starting graduate courses or certification in plastic surgery nursing. During the two years of basic surgical nursing, student nurses learn plastic surgery fundamentals from ASPSN introduction courses, core curriculum materials, and seminars pertaining to plastic surgery education, procedures, and issues.

The list on page 6 provides an overview of the minimum requirements for plastic surgery nursing.

Roles of Plastic Surgery Nurses

The roles of the plastic surgery nurse derive from the professional development of specific standards of care, required educational guidelines, and practice environments and settings for the plastic surgery patient.

The content in this appendix is not current and is of historical significance only.

Media coverage has deluged our society with information about plastic surgery that is often questionable, confusing the general public about its seriousness and providing economic incentives for physicians. Both the increasing awareness in our society (accurate and otherwise) of plastic surgery and the ambiguities of cosmetic surgery call for more nursing, consumer, and patient education interventions by plastic surgery nurses to help clarify misconceptions.

Minimum Requirements for Plastic Surgery Nursing

- Licensure as a registered nurse (RN) within the designated state of practice

- Education:
  - Minimum requirement—Associate degree from an accredited college of nursing
  - Preferred—Bachelor of Science degree in nursing from an accredited college of nursing

- Advanced knowledge in surgical principles, anatomy, and physiology for a specified age group (neonate, child, adolescent, adult, geriatric)

- Advanced knowledge in one or more of the following:
  - Wound care, burns, trauma, cancer-related disfigurements
  - Scar management, body image, health assessment, nutrition

- Continuing education and knowledge of current plastic surgery trends, issues, and procedures

- Certification—Registered nurses can earn specialty certification in plastic surgery nursing by meeting eligiblity requirements and passing the CPSN exam. A registered nurse must have two or more years experience working in plastic surgery nursing to become eligible to take the CPSN exam. The CPSN exam is a method to test and validate the skills, knowledge, and ability of the plastic surgery nurse. The Plastic Surgical Nursing Certification Board, comprised of registered nurses with content expertise in plastic surgery nursing, has oversight of the CPSN exam and collaborates and participates with other specialty nursing certifying bodies through the National Specialty Nursing Certifying Organization (NSNCO) in addressing issues related to certification, licensure, education, and research. Certification is suggested but not required.

The content in this appendix is not current and is of historical significance only.

One of the goals of plastic surgery nursing is to reach and educate other nurses and nursing students about plastic surgery issues, procedures, and current trends. Communication and interaction with other nursing specialties about the role of plastic surgery nurses will provide a broader understanding and knowledge base for nursing collaboration. Plastic surgery nurses help build the foundations of knowledge and education for improved outcomes, safety, health maintenance, and health awareness. It is through education and research that the practice of plastic surgery nursing can be recognized as a specialty.

General Nursing Role

Associate or bachelor degree nurses beginning clinical practice in their first year of licensure are encouraged to gain knowledge and develop skill levels associated with basic surgical principles in preparation for later specialization in plastic surgery nursing. Registered nurses who enter the field of plastic surgery must have a well-rounded knowledge base about various patient populations. The scope of knowledge required for the plastic surgery nurse varies with the area of practice interest, previous nursing experience, and level of educational preparation. The general level plastic surgery nurse will progress into a more expert role with experience, training, and additional education, which may include preparation for plastic surgery nursing subspecialties such as neonatal, pediatrics, general surgery, neurosurgery, advanced wound management, dermatology, burns, cancer, trauma, and operating room environments.

Advanced Practice Role

Advanced practice plastic surgery nursing roles are increasing in reaction to personal, professional, and societal needs. Nurse practitioner (NP) and clinical nurse specialist (CNS) are two of the roles included under the role of *advanced practice nurse* (*APN*) or *advanced practice registered nurse* (*APRN*). The advanced practice plastic surgery nurse is a registered nurse with a master's or higher degree in nursing. Credentialing is available for the CNS or NP advanced practice nurse in the specialty of plastic surgery.

Advanced practice registered nurses play a significant role in meeting the needs of the plastic surgery patient. Advanced practice nurses in plastic surgery are valuable to a practice because of their ability to use independent judgment in clinical decision-making, and to provide skilled, quality, and detailed advanced nursing care across the continuum. An advanced practice nurse in plastic surgery has the knowledge and training to provide comprehensive health assessments, differential diagnoses, and treatments for plastic surgery patients and others. Advanced practice nurses in plastic surgery advocate health maintenance, health promotion, and wellness.

Advanced practice nurses in plastic surgery serve as resources and consultants to other healthcare disciplines. The advanced practice nurse is instrumental in facilitating and conducting research in plastic surgery. The advanced practice nurse also plays a key role in providing continuity of care for the plastic surgery patient. Legislation has now made prescriptive authority and third-party reimbursement possible for the advanced practice nurse in the plastic surgery arena. The roles of the advanced practice nurse in plastic surgery are developing and expanding. National certification in advanced practice plastic surgery nursing is recommended. Many advanced practice nurses in plastic surgery have advanced practice certifications in other areas.

Educator Role

As the need for plastic surgery education becomes more evident, so is the need to disseminate education throughout the nursing field and the general population. Nurse educators promote educational clarity, standards, knowledge, and safety related to plastic surgery procedures, issues, and outcomes. In this document, the plastic surgery nurse in an educator role will be referred to as the *plastic surgery nurse educator*.

A plastic surgery nurse educator is educated at the bachelor, graduate, or doctorate degree level with a focus on plastic surgery education. Plastic surgery nurse educators also comply with and support state educational requirements to teach at community or university institutions according to their educational background. At the graduate or doctoral level, the plastic surgery nurse educator has the opportunity to facilitate and develop focused education, curriculums, and research in plastic surgery.

A plastic surgery nurse educator develops instruction, guidelines, materials, and programs for nurses during nursing school rotations, distant learning experiences, and in various practices, environments, and settings related to plastic surgery. A plastic surgery nurse educator also provides education for local and national communities on plastic surgery and relevant resources.

A plastic surgery nurse educator conducts a needs assessment to help establish educational requirements in various practice environments and settings. A plastic surgery nurse educator functions as an educator and a liaison between the plastic surgeon or advanced practice plastic surgery nurse and the patient to help ensure continuity of care, health promotion, and health maintenance. Providing educational materials during the consultation, preoperative, and postoperative stages is key to educational consistency among staff members, plastic surgeons, advanced practice plastic surgery nurses, and plastic surgery patients. A plastic surgery nurse educator provides an appropriate climate for learning, and ensures that the learners are actively involved in the learning process and in identification of learning outcomes through in-service updates on current issues, procedures, or products related to plastic surgery. Plastic surgery nurse educators evaluate the effectiveness and outcomes of various educational strategies and then provide a revised plan to correct any shortcomings.

A plastic surgery nurse educator is a member of a multidisciplinary team, and functions as a consultant, change agent, leader, and resource to other nursing and healthcare disciplines. Plastic surgery nurse educators help to conduct research and disseminate findings. A plastic surgery nurse educator requires a strong knowledge base of teaching and learning theories, curriculum development, research, test and measurement evaluation methods, critical thinking skills, and quality improvement techniques.

Plastic Surgery Nursing Research

Research is a group of activities designed to expand knowledge. Research includes utilization of theories, principles, or relationships. Research helps to streamline or reorganize existing bodies of information, to verify existing theory, and to apply existing knowledge.

Both reconstructive and aesthetic surgical outcomes need to be evaluated and assessed for improved patient outcomes and health management. In order to introduce new materials, refine educational guidelines, and provide valid evidence to support or discard current practice regimens, nursing research is crucial. Nurses must demonstrate scientifically that nursing interventions make a positive difference in the outcomes and health status of plastic surgery patients. Nurses need research-based knowledge to improve decision-making skills regarding proper care for plastic surgery patients and to implement and evaluate care management. Because of the psychological and clinical aspects of plastic surgery, both the qualitative and quantitative approaches to research can be used to evaluate plastic surgery research criteria and outcomes.

Through the translation and dissemination of research, nursing will continue as an independent professional entity in health care, fulfilling its responsibility in collegial relationships with other professionals. Application of research findings in practice is important to improve patient outcomes and quality of life, enhance nursing practice, and deliver effective, quality health care. The current research of nursing professionals is building a solid theoretical foundation for the plastic surgery nursing practice of the future. Topics of plastic surgery nursing research include nursing strategies different from the activities and actions of other disciplines, outcome measures, program evaluation, nursing interventions, and historical issues of ethics and policy. Knowledge of plastic surgery nursing research is needed to enhance the professional practice of all nurses, including both consumers of research (those who read, evaluate, and implement practice-based changes from studies) and producers (those who undertake research studies).

Practice Environments and Settings for the Plastic Surgery Nurse

The plastic surgery nurse provides care for patients and their families or caretakers in a variety of settings and locations that include hospitals, outpatient ambulatory surgery centers, office-based surgery centers, and private practice. The plastic surgery nurse is prepared to educate and provide comprehensive care to patients in a safe and regulated environment. The plastic surgery nurse provides competent, ethical, and appropriate nursing care to help improve surgical experiences and outcomes. In order to determine and implement the plan of care, and to ensure optimal outcomes for the plastic surgery patient, the plastic surgery nurse encourages and facilitates consultations, communication, and collaboration with other healthcare team members.

Plastic surgery nurses are also knowledgeable of proper policies, procedures, contracts, and regulations, including those for compliance with the Health Insurance Portability and Accountability Act (HIPAA), in appropriate and designated plastic surgery settings. Plastic surgery nurses know and comply with the requirements for federal, state, local, insurance, and accreditation agency standards. Plastic surgery nurses help promote safer surgical services for the plastic surgery patient.

Hospital

The plastic surgery nurse working in the hospital environment may care for plastic surgery patients in a variety of specialty departments or units. These include, among others, emergency departments, operating rooms, surgical floor/units, burn units, critical care units, neonatal units, pediatrics, and oncology. Plastic surgery nursing within the hospital environment is multidimensional and includes skills, functions, roles, and responsibilities that evolve from the body of knowledge specific to plastic surgery nursing. These dimensions are apparent in the plastic surgery nursing roles, processes, and characteristics. The plastic surgery nurse practicing in the hospital environment may provide assessment, analysis, nursing diagnosis, planning, implementation of interventions, outcome identification, and evaluation of patients in all age groups whose care requires plastic surgery interventions, procedures, and/or treatments. Regulatory factors pertinent to plastic surgery nurses working in the hospital environment include the Joint Commission on Accreditation of Healthcare Organizations (JCAHO); specific hospital rules and regulations; and rules, regulations, and guidelines governed by each state board of nursing that ensure public safety.

Outpatient /Ambulatory Surgery Center

The plastic surgery nurse working in the outpatient/ambulatory surgery center demonstrates the appropriate skills, knowledge, competencies, and abilities to provide proper and safe nursing care for the plastic surgery patient in the preoperative, operative, and postoperative stages of the plastic surgery procedure. The outpatient/ambulatory surgery center must be accredited or certified by the appropriate surgery center accreditation for the state where the plastic surgery nurse holds a license.

The plastic surgery nurse functions within the guidelines of the Accreditation Association for Ambulatory Health Care (AAAHC), the AAAHC Institute for Quality Improvement (IQI), and the American Association

The content in this appendix is not current and is of historical significance only.

for Accreditation of Ambulatory Surgery Facilities (AAAASF). The plastic surgery nurse promotes higher quality surgical outcomes by maintaining standards, measuring performance, and providing consultation and education. The plastic surgery nurse complies with and promotes the laws and regulations governing the operation of the facility, such as Occupational Safety and Health Administration (OSHA) standards for bloodborne pathogens and hazardous waste; the Americans with Disabilities Act; and appropriate federal, state, and local laws. The plastic surgery nurse working in an outpatient/ambulatory surgery center maintains the plastic surgery nursing standards of practice and standards of professional performance.

Office-Based Surgery Center

According to ASPS (2004) statistical data, 56% of aesthetic plastic surgery procedures and 51% of reconstructive plastic surgery procedures are performed in a plastic surgeon's office. This poses risks if the office does not have a properly accredited or regulated surgery facility. Public awareness and understanding of proper accreditation and regulation are needed to provide clarity and guidance when considering plastic surgery. The plastic surgery nurse is aware of the potential confusion surrounding office-based surgery and can be instrumental in providing proper education about accreditation and regulation for other nurses, patients, and communities. The plastic surgery nurse working in an office-based surgery center demonstrates the appropriate skills, knowledge, competencies, and abilities to provide proper nursing care for the plastic surgery patient.

The plastic surgery nurse's role in the office-based surgery center includes the consultation, preoperative, postoperative, and follow-up stages of the plastic surgery procedure. Assessment, education, planning and intervention are part of the plastic surgery nurse's role during each stage of a plastic surgery procedure. The plastic surgery nurse helps to improve the quality of care by maintaining standards, including the Standards of Plastic Surgery Nursing, measuring performance, and providing education within the specific office-based surgery center.

The plastic surgery nurse working in the office-based surgery center complies with, and promotes compliance with, the laws and regulations governing the operation of the office-based surgery facility, such as the OSHA standards for bloodborne pathogens and hazardous waste; the

Americans with Disabilities Act; and appropriate federal, state, and local laws. The plastic surgery nurse should also know and address compliance with the guidelines of the Accreditation Association for Ambulatory Health Care (AAAHC), the AAAHC Institute for Quality Improvement (IQI) and the American Association for Accreditation of Ambulatory Surgery Facilities, Inc. (AAAASF).

Private Practice

The private practice setting provides plastic surgery nurses with the opportunity to interact directly with the patient throughout the plastic surgery process and recovery. Mutual goals and surgical expectations are assessed on a more personal and interactive level than other settings. Preoperative and postoperative evaluations are more accessible and can provide valuable information when evaluating quality of outcomes. The plastic surgery nurse in private practice is encouraged to have two or more years of plastic surgery nurse experience within a hospital or outpatient/ambulatory surgery center. The plastic surgery nurse in private practice requires competence and confidence to respond appropriately and safely to plastic surgery patients and their needs.

The plastic surgery nurse working in a physician-owned and -supervised private practice may possess an associate degree or higher, and function quite like an advanced practice nurse or nurse educator in the practice environment. Responsibilities may include assessment of an individual patient's needs, educational material development, assisting physicians or advanced practice plastic surgery nurses, staff education, and in-service and patient education. The plastic surgery nurse assesses educational needs and then provides educational material and instruction on the plastic surgery procedure.

The plastic surgery nurse also provides preoperative and postoperative counseling regarding technical aspects of the surgical procedure, documented health assessment, pertinent mutual goal planning, and psychosocial assessment and support. The plastic surgery nurse may provide consumer education about selecting an appropriate plastic surgery facility and provider that will meet the patient's needs and provide the best outcomes. The plastic surgery nurse in private practice provides follow-up communication and evaluation to ensure quality of care, health maintenance, and proper documentation for the plastic

The content in this appendix is not current and is of historical significance only.

surgery patient. The plastic surgery nurse in private practice maintains the plastic surgery nursing standards of practice and standards of professional performance.

Patient Population

The plastic surgery nurse interacts with and cares for patients who require or desire plastic or reconstructive surgery for enhancement or restoration purposes. The plastic surgery nurse also interacts with and educates families of plastic surgery patients, as well as communities, regarding plastic surgery procedures and issues. The plastic surgery nurse has the special knowledge and skills needed to meet the needs of the patient population. The plastic surgery nurse provides care for patients in a variety of settings, age groups, and populations, including neonatal, pediatric, adult, geriatric, general surgery, neurosurgery, advanced wound management, dermatology, burns, cancer, and trauma patients.

Patients receiving care and education from a plastic surgery nurse require a thorough understanding of procedures, personal expectations, and mutual goal setting in order to achieve maximum satisfaction and health maintenance. Plastic surgery nurses help patients to deal with perceived or altered body image, perceived surgical outcomes, fears, and learning needs associated with a surgical intervention. Patients undergoing plastic surgery may encounter psychological, emotional, and physical imbalances during the recovery phase. Managing the psychological discord associated with physical alterations requires specialized knowledge and education.

Reconstructive Plastic Surgery Patient Population

Reconstructive plastic surgery includes skin, breast, trunk, craniomaxillofacial structures, musculoskeletal system, extremities, and external genitalia. Nurses in reconstructive plastic surgery require specialized knowledge related to complex wounds, replantation, grafts, flaps, free tissue transfer, and use of implantable materials reconstruction or repair due to cancer, trauma, burns, superficial injury, congenital defects, or disease. Plastic surgery nurses help the patient to express psychological, physical, and psychosocial needs in order to regain or rediscover coping strategies and successful interaction with society. Thorough assessment and documentation before, during, and after surgery is essential for proper evaluation of patient outcomes.

Aesthetic Plastic Surgery Patient Population

Aesthetic plastic surgery includes skin, breast, trunk, craniomaxillofacial structures, musculoskeletal system, extremities, and external genitalia. Aesthetic plastic surgery may be performed after reconstructive surgery to improve overall results. Plastic surgery nurses require specialized knowledge associated with reconstructive surgical principles to assist in the successful recovery and outcomes of the aesthetic surgery patient. Aesthetic surgery includes adjustment, enhancement, and alteration according to each patient's request for plastic surgery intervention. Thorough assessment and documentation before, during, and after surgery is essential for proper evaluation of patient outcomes.

Ethics and Advocacy in Plastic Surgery Nursing

Ethics is a fundamental part of nursing. Ethical awareness, judgments, and decisions are founded on a combination of principles, theories, and moral foundations. Nursing ethics are based on care and the actions of caring, to enhance and protect patient well-being. Plastic surgery nurses are expected to comply with and promote the ethical ideals, model, code, and principles of the nursing profession. *Code of Ethics for Nurses with Interpretive Statements* (ANA 2001) is the framework on which plastic surgery nurses base ethical analysis and decision-making, and on which standards are based. The plastic surgery nurse is also an advocate for the patient and provides care in a non-discriminatory and non-judgmental way. Patient advocacy means preservation of patient autonomy, execution of clinical judgments, and management of ethical issues.

The plastic surgery nurse maintains the plastic surgery standards of practice and standards of professional performance in each type of practice environment to help ensure the safety, quality of care, and the highest level of health maintenance or health restoration for the plastic surgery patient. The plastic surgery nurse promotes an ethical practice environment by serving as a patient advocate. The plastic surgery nurse's attitude and performance reflect compassion and understanding of a patient's self-respect, cultural beliefs, sovereignty, and rights to self-

The content in this appendix is not current and is of historical significance only.

determination and privacy. Plastic surgery nurses implement the principles of autonomy, nonmaleficence, beneficence, and justice when interacting with patients requiring or desiring plastic surgery intervention. Plastic surgery nurses are aware of the many ethical considerations associated with plastic surgery. These include misleading advertising, the aging population, insurance reimbursement, and other matters. Public awareness of these issues is key to proper acknowledgment of the physical and emotional health risks of plastic surgery.

Misleading Advertising

Advertisements for plastic surgery are found on the Internet, television, magazines, and radio. Many plastic or cosmetic surgery advertisements do not disclose risks, recovery time, contraindications, physician credentials, type of board certification, or type of surgical facility. Plastic surgery nurses encourage consumers interested in plastic surgery to inquire about the physician, the surgical environment, and the procedure in detail in order make an informed decision. The ABPS (2003) does not approve of plastic surgery advertising that raises unrealistic, false, or misleading expectations. Public awareness of advertising statements that minimize risks is one goal of plastic surgery nursing in its community education campaigns.

The Aging Population

The quest for a more youthful appearance to complement longevity is spreading among the aging population in our society. Aging adults are considered vulnerable because of age-related physical and cognitive changes that make them more susceptible to health risks during and after surgery. According to the ASPS statistical chart for age distribution (2004), aesthetic plastic surgery procedures for ages 65 and over increased 5 from 2002 to 2003. Over 400,000 aesthetic plastic surgery procedures were performed on patients 65 and older in 2003. Plastic surgery nurses must be aware of the specialized needs of the aging population, as well as the ethical considerations associated with aesthetic surgery requests by patients. Opportunities for plastic surgery nurses to serve as patient advocates for the aging population are increasing as the demand for aesthetic surgery procedures and treatments increases.

Insurance Reimbursements

The ethics of insurance reimbursements for plastic surgery procedures is still controversial. The question centers around how insurance companies view reconstructive vs. aesthetic surgery. Reconstructive plastic surgery may be needed as a result of cancer, trauma, burns, superficial injury, congenital defects, or disease. Aesthetic plastic surgery may then follow reconstructive plastic surgery in order to improve results. Insurance reimbursements may not be granted for those requiring multiple surgeries for the best possible outcomes. A plastic surgery nurse in a plastic surgery practice environment may act as a patient advocate or a change agent to help improve insurance reimbursements.

The content in this appendix is not current and is of historical significance only.

STANDARDS OF PLASTIC SURGERY NURSING PRACTICE
STANDARDS OF PRACTICE

All plastic surgery nursing practice standards and documentation will abide by current statutes, rules, regulations, and the guidelines of the Health Insurance Portability and Accountability Act (HIPAA).

STANDARD 1. ASSESSMENT

The plastic surgery nurse collects comprehensive data pertinent to the patient's health or the situation.

Measurement Criteria:

The plastic surgery nurse:

- Collects data in a systematic and ongoing process.
- Includes the patient, family, significant others, and appropriate healthcare providers in the holistic data collection process.
- Records pertinent data in the patient's permanent medical record,
- Is sensitive to cultural diversity, ethnicity, gender, and lifestyle choices.
- Prioritizes data collection according to the patient's immediate health condition, or the anticipated needs of the plastic surgery patient or situation.
- Uses appropriate evidence-based assessment techniques and instruments in collecting pertinent data.
- Uses analytical models and problem-solving tools.
- Synthesizes available data, information, and knowledge relevant to the situation to identify patterns and variances.
- Documents relevant data in a retrievable format.

Additional Measurement Criteria for the Advanced Practice Registered Nurse:

The advanced practice registered nurse in plastic surgery:

- Conducts in-depth and comprehensive assessments based on a synthesis of individual and family health.

Continued ▶

- Bases assessments on advanced knowledge in the field of plastic surgery.

- Initiates and interprets diagnostic tests and procedures relevant to the current status of plastic surgery patient.

The content in this appendix is not current and is of historical significance only.

Standard 2. Diagnosis

The plastic surgery nurse analyzes the assessment data to determine the diagnosis or issues.

Measurement Criteria:

The plastic surgery nurse:

- Derives the diagnosis and issues from the assessment data obtained during interview, physical examination, diagnostic test, or diagnostic procedures.

- Bases the diagnosis on actual or potential responses to alterations in health.

- Discusses and validates the diagnoses or issues with the plastic surgery patient, significant others, and other appropriate healthcare providers when possible.

- Documents the diagnosis or issues, and communicates them in a manner that facilitates the plan of care, interventions, expected outcomes, and plan for the plastic surgery patient.

Additional Measurement Criteria for the Advanced Practice Registered Nurse:

The advanced practice registered nurse in plastic surgery:

- Systematically compares and contrasts clinical findings of the plastic surgery patient with normal and abnormal variations and developmental events when formulating a differential diagnosis.

- Utilizes complex data and information obtained during interview, examination, and diagnostic procedures, and initiates further appropriate diagnostic tests to complete the diagnostic analysis.

- Assists staff in building and sustaining competency in the diagnostic process.

STANDARD 3. OUTCOMES IDENTIFICATION

The plastic surgery nurse identifies expected outcomes individualized to the patient or the situation.

Measurement Criteria:

The plastic surgery nurse:

- Jointly formulates expected plastic surgery patient outcomes with input from the plastic surgery patient, family, significant others, and healthcare providers when possible and appropriate.

- Derives culturally appropriate expected outcomes from the diagnoses.

- Considers available resources, associated risks, benefits, costs, current scientific evidence, and clinical expertise when developing expected outcomes of the plastic surgery patient.

- Determines expected outcomes with reflection and sensitivity to the plastic surgery patient, the patient's values, ethical considerations, environment or situation, cultural diversity, ethnicity, gender, and lifestyle choices.

- Determines expected outcomes with consideration of associated risks, benefits, costs, and current scientific evidence.

- Includes a time estimate for attainment of expected outcomes.

- Develops expected outcomes that realistically consider the plastic surgery patient's current and potential physical capabilities and provide direction for continuity of care.

- Modifies expected outcomes based on changes in the status of the plastic surgery patient or evaluation of the situation.

- Documents expected outcomes as measurable goals.

Additional Measurement Criteria for the Advanced Practice Registered Nurse:

The advanced practice registered nurse in plastic surgery:

- Identifies expected outcomes that include scientific evidence and are attainable through implementation of evidence-based practices.

- Identifies expected outcomes that incorporate cost and clinical effectiveness, patient satisfaction, and continuity and consistency among providers.

The content in this appendix is not current and is of historical significance only.

- Supports the use of clinical guidelines associated with positive plastic surgery patient outcomes.

- Modifies expected outcomes based on changes in the plastic surgery patient's or family's health status.

The content in this appendix is not current and is of historical significance only.

STANDARD 4. PLANNING

The plastic surgery nurse develops a plan of care that prescribes strategies and alternatives to attain expected outcomes.

Measurement Criteria:

The plastic surgery nurse:

- Individualizes the plan of care to the physical, emotional, psycho-social, cultural, and spiritual needs, desires, and resources of the plastic surgery patient and family.

- Develops the plan of care in collaboration with the plastic surgery patient, family, and other healthcare providers as appropriate.

- Documents strategies in the plan appropriate to each of the identified diagnoses or issues, and that may include strategies for health promotion, disease prevention, and restoration of health for the plastic surgery patient.

- Provides for continuity of care in the plan.

- Integrates an implementation pathway or timeline within the plan.

- Institutes the plan priorities with the plastic surgery patient, family, and others as appropriate.

- Uses the plan to guide treatment of the plastic surgery patient by other members of the healthcare team.

- Defines the plan that reflects current state laws, policies, regulations, and standards.

- Integrates current trends and scientific research in the planning process.

- Considers the economic impact of the plan on the plastic surgery patient.

- Utilizes standardized language or recognized terminology to record the plan.

Additional Measurement Criteria for the Advanced Practice Registered Nurse:

The advanced practice registered nurse in plastic surgery:

- Identifies assessment, diagnostic strategies, and therapeutic interventions in the plan that reflect current evidence, including data, research, literature, and expert clinical knowledge.

- Selects or designs strategies to meet the multifaceted needs of complex plastic surgery patients.

- Includes the synthesis of the plastic surgery patient's values and beliefs regarding nursing and medical therapies within the plan.

The content in this appendix is not current and is of historical significance only.

STANDARD 5. IMPLEMENTATION

The plastic surgery nurse implements the identified plan of care.

Measurement Criteria:

The plastic surgery nurse:

- Implements the plan of care for the plastic surgery patient in a safe and timely manner.

- Documents implementation of the plan, including any changes to or omissions from the plan.

- Employs evidence-based interventions and treatments for the plastic surgery patient that are relevant to the diagnosis or problem.

- Selects and implements interventions based on available community resources and systems.

- Collaborates with other appropriate members of the interdisciplinary healthcare team to implement the plan of care for the plastic surgery patient.

Additional Measurement Criteria for the Advanced Practice Registered Nurse:

The advanced practice registered nurse in plastic surgery:

- Facilitates in the utilization of systems and community resources to implement the plan of care for the plastic surgery patient.

- Supports the collaboration with other appropriate members of the interdisciplinary healthcare team to implement the plan of care for the plastic surgery patient.

- Incorporates new information, data, and strategies to initiate change in nursing care practices if preferred outcomes are not achieved.

STANDARD 5A: COORDINATION OF CARE

The plastic surgery nurse coordinates care delivery.

Measurement Criteria:

The plastic surgery nurse:

- Coordinates implementation of the plan of care.

- Documents the coordination of the care and treatments.

Additional Measurement Criteria for the Advanced Practice Registered Nurse:

The advanced practice registered nurse in plastic surgery:

- Provides leadership in the coordination of multidisciplinary health care for integrated delivery of patient care services.

- Synthesizes data and information to recommend necessary system and community support measures, including any environmental adjustments.

- Coordinates system and community resources that enhance delivery of care across continuums.

- Considers the plastic surgery patient's and family's complex needs and desired outcomes when coordinating and negotiating health-related and other specialized care needs.

The content in this appendix is not current and is of historical significance only.

STANDARD 5B: HEALTH TEACHING AND HEALTH PROMOTION

The plastic surgery nurse employs strategies to promote health and a safe environment.

Measurement Criteria:

The plastic surgery nurse:

- Provides education in such topics as healthy lifestyles, risk-reducing behaviors, developmental needs, activities of daily living, and preventive self-care.

- Promotes quality of life for the plastic surgery patient and family members by maximizing, restoring, and maintaining functional status to promote activities of daily living, as appropriate to the plastic surgery patient and the improvement of their safety and welfare.

- Utilizes health promotion and health teaching methods appropriate to the situation, and that recognize developmental level, culture, learning needs, readiness and ability to learn, language preference, and other factors of the plastic surgery patient and the family.

- Seeks opportunities for feedback and evaluation of the effectiveness of the strategies and interventions used.

Additional Measurement Criteria for the Advanced Practice Registered Nurse:

The advanced practice registered nurse in plastic surgery:

- Synthesizes empirical evidence on risk behaviors, learning theories, behavioral change theories, motivational theories, epidemiology, and other related theories and frameworks when designing health information and patient education.

- Designs health information and patient education appropriate to the plastic surgery patient's developmental level, learning needs, health, cultural beliefs and practices, and readiness to learn.

- Evaluates health information resources, such as the Internet and peer-reviewed journals, within the area of plastic surgery for accuracy, readability, and comprehensibility to help plastic surgery patients access quality health information.

STANDARD 5C: CONSULTATION

The advanced practice registered nurse in plastic surgery provides consultation to influence the specified plan, enhance the abilities of others, and effect change.

Measurement Criteria for the Advanced Practice Registered Nurse:

The advanced practice registered nurse in plastic surgery:

- Synthesizes clinical data, theoretical frameworks, and evidence when providing consultation.

- Facilitates the effectiveness of a consultation by involving the plastic surgery patient and other stakeholders in the decision-making process.

- Communicates consultation recommendations that facilitate change.

The content in this appendix is not current and is of historical significance only.

STANDARD 5D: PRESCRIPTIVE AUTHORITY AND TREATMENT

The advanced practice registered nurse in plastic surgery uses prescriptive authority, procedures, referrals, treatments, and therapies in accordance with state and federal laws and regulations.

Measurement Criteria for the Advanced Practice Registered Nurse:

The advanced practice registered nurse in plastic surgery:

- Prescribes evidence-based treatments, therapies, and procedures for the plastic surgery patient after considering the patient's complete healthcare needs.

- Prescribes pharmacologic agents based on current knowledge and information of pharmacology and physiology.

- Prescribes specific pharmacological agents and/or treatments based on clinical indicators, the plastic surgery patient's status and needs, and the results of diagnostic and laboratory tests.

- Evaluates therapeutic and potential adverse effects of pharmacological and non-pharmacological treatments.

- Provides plastic surgery patients with information about intended effects and potential adverse effects of proposed prescriptive therapies.

- Provides information to the plastic surgery patient about costs, and alternative treatments and procedures, as appropriate.

STANDARD 6: EVALUATION

The plastic surgery nurse evaluates the patient's progress towards achievement of outcomes.

Measurement Criteria:

The plastic surgery registered nurse:

- Conducts a systematic, ongoing, and criterion-based evaluation of the outcomes for the plastic surgery patient in relation to the structures and processes prescribed by the plan and the indicated timeline.

- Includes the plastic surgery patient, appropriate members of the interdisciplinary healthcare team, and others involved in the care or situation in the evaluative process.

- Evaluates the effectiveness of the planned strategies and interventions in relation to the plastic surgery patient's responses and the attainment of the expected outcomes.

- Documents the results of the evaluation.

- Utilizes ongoing assessment data to revise or resolve the diagnoses, the outcomes, the plan of care, and the implementation as needed.

- Disseminates the results of the evaluation to the plastic surgery patient and others involved in the care or situation, as appropriate, in accordance with state and federal laws and regulations.

Additional Measurement Criteria for the Advanced Practice Registered Nurse:

The advanced practice registered nurse in plastic surgery:

- Evaluates the accuracy of the diagnosis and effectiveness of the interventions in relationship to the plastic surgery patient's attainment of expected outcomes.

- Incorporates advanced knowledge, practice, and research into the evaluation process.

- Synthesizes the results of the evaluation analyses to determine the impact of the plan on the affected plastic surgery patients, families, groups, communities, and institutions.

Continued ▶

The content in this appendix is not current and is of historical significance only.

- Uses the results of the evaluation analyses to make or recommend process or structural changes, including policy, procedure, or protocol documentation, as appropriate.

The content in this appendix is not current and is of historical significance only.

STANDARDS OF PROFESSIONAL PERFORMANCE

STANDARD 7. QUALITY OF PRACTICE

The plastic surgery nurse systematically strengthens the quality and effectiveness of nursing practice.

Measurement Criteria:

The plastic surgery nurse:

- Demonstrates quality by documenting the application of the nursing process in a responsible, accountable, and ethical manner.

- Uses the results of quality improvement activities to initiate change in nursing practice and in the healthcare delivery system.

- Uses creativity and innovation in nursing practice to improve care delivery for the plastic surgery patient.

- Incorporates new knowledge to initiate changes in nursing practice if desired outcomes are not achieved.

- Participates in quality improvement activities as appropriate to the nurse's position, education, and practice environment. Activities may include:

  - Identifying aspects of practice important for quality monitoring.

  - Developing indicators that are utilized to monitor the quality and effectiveness of plastic surgery nursing professional practice.

  - Collecting data to monitor quality and effectiveness of plastic surgery nursing practice.

  - Analyzing quality improvement data to recognize opportunities to improve plastic surgery nursing practice.

  - Formulating recommendations to improve plastic surgery nursing care or plastic surgery patient outcomes.

  - Implementing activities to strengthen the quality of nursing practice for the plastic surgery patient.

  - Developing, implementing, and evaluating policies, procedures, and practice guidelines to improve the quality of practice.

  - Participating on multidisciplinary teams to evaluate clinical practice or health services.

Continued ▶

The content in this appendix is not current and is of historical significance only.

- Taking part in efforts to decrease or minimize costs and redundancy.

- Analyzing factors related to safety and satisfaction, and cost–benefit options associated with quality and effectiveness.

- Analyzing organizational systems for barriers.

- Implementing processes to decrease or remove barriers within organizational systems.

Additional Measurement Criteria for the Advanced Practice Registered Nurse:

The advanced practice registered nurse in plastic surgery:

- Obtains and maintains professional certification in plastic surgery nursing.

- Designs quality improvement initiatives.

- Implements initiatives to evaluate the need for change.

- Evaluates the plastic surgery practice environment and the quality of nursing care using existing evidence, and identifies opportunities for the generation and use of research.

STANDARD 8. EDUCATION

The plastic surgery nurse attains knowledge and competency that reflects current plastic surgery nursing practice.

Measurement Criteria:

The plastic surgery nurse:

- Participates in ongoing educational activities related to practice knowledge and professional issues.

- Demonstrates a commitment to lifelong learning through self-reflection and inquiry to identify learning needs.

- Seeks experiences that reflect current plastic surgery practice in order to develop, maintain, or refine clinical competence or role performance in plastic surgery.

- Acquires knowledge and skills appropriate to the plastic surgery setting, role, or situation by participating in educational programs and activities, conferences, workshops, and interdisciplinary professional meetings.

- Documents and maintains professional records that provide evidence of educational activities, competencies, and lifelong learning.

- Actively and regularly seeks formal and independent learning experiences and opportunities that will advance the nurse's knowledge in plastic surgery, and that meet established goals for professional development.

Additional Measurement Criteria for the Advanced Practice Registered Nurse:

The advanced practice registered nurse in plastic surgery:

- Utilizes current healthcare research findings, scientific findings, and other evidence to expand clinical knowledge, enhance role performance, and increase knowledge of professional issues.

STANDARD 9. PROFESSIONAL PRACTICE EVALUATION

The plastic surgery nurse evaluates one's own nursing practice in relation to professional practice standards and guidelines, relevant statutes, rules, and regulations.

Measurement Criteria:

The plastic surgery nurse's practice reflects the application of knowledge of current practice standards, guidelines, statutes, rules, and regulations.

The plastic surgery nurse:

- Provides age-appropriate care in a culturally and ethnically sensitive manner.

- Engages in a personal performance evaluation on a regular basis, identifying areas of strengths as well as areas in which professional practice development would be beneficial.

- Participates in and seeks informal feedback regarding their own nursing practice and role performance from plastic surgery patients, peers, professional colleagues, and others.

- Participates in systematic peer review as appropriate.

- Takes action to achieve the professional development goals recognized during ongoing and formal performance evaluations.

- Provides rationales for practice beliefs, decisions, and actions as part of the informal and formal evaluation process.

Additional Measurement Criteria for the Advanced Practice Registered Nurse:

The advanced practice registered nurse in plastic surgery:

- Engages in a formal process seeking feedback regarding their own practice from patients, peers, professional colleagues, and others.

STANDARD 10. COLLEGIALITY

The plastic surgery nurse interacts with and contributes to the professional development of peers, colleagues, and other healthcare providers.

Measurement Criteria:

The plastic surgery nurse:

- Shares knowledge, expertise, clinical observations, and skills with peers, colleagues, and other healthcare team members as evidenced by such activities as plastic surgery patient care conferences or presentations at formal or informal meetings.

- Provides peers with constructive feedback regarding their practice and/or role performance.

- Interacts with peers and colleagues to enhance one's own professional nursing practice and/or role performance.

- Contributes to and maintains a supportive and healthy work environment that fosters compassionate and caring relationships with peers and colleagues.

- Contributes to the learning experiences and education of healthcare providers, students, and others through role modeling, acting as a resource, mentoring, or serving as a preceptor or instructor in the plastic surgery clinical setting.

- Differentiates the scope and function of each member of the interdisciplinary healthcare team caring for the plastic surgery patient.

- Contributes to a supportive and healthy plastic surgery work environment.

Additional Measurement Criteria for the Advanced Practice Registered Nurse:

The advanced practice registered nurse in plastic surgery:

- Demonstrates expert practice to interdisciplinary team members and healthcare consumers.

- Mentors and serves as a role model, preceptor, and facilitator of learning in generalist plastic surgery nursing care, in advanced practice plastic surgery nursing, and to other registered nurses and colleagues as appropriate.

Continued ▶

The content in this appendix is not current and is of historical significance only.

- Participates with interdisciplinary teams who contribute to role development and advanced nursing practice and health care.

- Serves as a liaison to institutional, local, state, and national legislative bodies in order to facilitate communication of issues regarding advanced practice in the plastic surgery arena.

STANDARD 11. COLLABORATION

The plastic surgery nurse collaborates with the plastic surgery patient, family, and others in the conduct of nursing practice.

Measurement Criteria:

The plastic surgery nurse:

- Communicates with the plastic surgery patient, family, members of the interdisciplinary healthcare team, and other healthcare providers regarding patient care and the nurse's role in providing that care.

- Collaborates in creating a documented plan focused on outcomes and decisions related to care and delivery of services for the plastic surgery patient, and indicating communication with the plastic surgery patient, family, and appropriate others.

- Coordinates the implementation of care provided for the plastic surgery patient and family by the interdisciplinary healthcare team.

- Partners with others to effect change and generate positive outcomes through knowledge of the plastic surgery patient or situation.

- Documents referrals, including provisions, for continuity of care.

Additional Measurement Criteria for the Advanced Practice Registered Nurse:

The advanced practice registered nurse in plastic surgery:

- Partners with other disciplines to enhance plastic surgery patient care through interdisciplinary activities, such as education, consultation, management, technological development, or research opportunities.

- Contributes to optimizing advanced practice nursing care for the plastic surgery patient in the areas of health education, health promotion, health restoration, and health maintenance.

- Promotes and facilitates an interdisciplinary healthcare process with other members of the healthcare team.

Continued ▶

- Participates in establishing plastic surgery nursing clinical practice guidelines, clinical pathways, and practice protocols.

- Documents the plastic surgery patient's plan of care communications, rationales for plan of care changes, and collaborative discussions to improve his or her care.

The content in this appendix is not current and is of historical significance only.

STANDARD 12. ETHICS

The plastic surgery nurse integrates ethical provisions in all areas of practice.

Measurement Criteria:

The plastic surgery nurse:

- Utilizes *Code of Ethics for Nurses with Interpretive Statements* (ANA 2001) to guide practice.

- Provides care for the plastic surgery patient in a manner that ensures that the plastic surgery patient's autonomy, dignity, and rights are preserved.

- Maintains plastic surgery patient privacy and confidentiality within legal and regulatory parameters.

- Acts as a patient advocate and liaison, assisting plastic surgery patients in developing skills for self-advocacy.

- Maintains a therapeutic and professional patient–nurse relationship with appropriate professional role boundaries.

- Demonstrates a commitment to practicing self-care, managing stress, and connecting with self and others.

- Recognizes one's own values and beliefs when assisting in the formulation of ethical decisions.

- Contributes to resolving the ethical problems or dilemmas of the plastic surgery patient, colleagues, or systems as evidenced in such activities as participating on ethics committees, and seeking available resources to help formulate ethical decisions.

- Reports abuse of the plastic surgery patient's rights, or illegal, incompetent, or impaired practices.

Additional Measurement Criteria for the Advanced Practice Registered Nurse:

The advanced practice registered nurse in plastic surgery:

- Informs the plastic surgery patient of the risks, benefits, and outcomes of healthcare regimens.

- Participates in interdisciplinary teams that address ethical risks, benefits, and outcomes for the plastic surgery patient.

STANDARD 13. RESEARCH

The plastic surgery nurse integrates research findings into practice.

Measurement Criteria:

The plastic surgery nurse:

- Utilizes the best available evidence, including research findings, to guide practice decisions for the plastic surgery patient.

- Actively participates in research activities at various levels as appropriate to the nurse's level of education and position. Activities may include:

  - Identifying clinical problems specific to nursing research such as patient care and nursing practice.

  - Participating in data collection such as surveys, pilot projects, and formal studies.

  - Participating in a formal committee or program.

  - Sharing research activities and/or findings with peers and others.

  - Conducting research.

  - Critically analyzing and interpreting research findings for application to plastic surgery practice.

  - Utilizing research findings to develop or initiate change in policies, procedures, and standards of practice in plastic surgery patient care.

  - Incorporating research as a basis for learning.

Additional Measurement Criteria for the Advanced Practice Registered Nurse:

The advanced practice registered nurse in plastic surgery:

- Contributes to plastic surgery nursing knowledge by conducting or synthesizing research that discovers, examines, and evaluates knowledge, theories, criteria, and creative approaches to improve healthcare practice for the plastic surgery patient.

- Formally disseminates research findings through activities such as presentations, publications, consultation, and journal clubs.

STANDARD 14. RESOURCE UTILIZATION

The plastic surgery nurse considers factors related to safety, effectiveness, cost, and impact on practice in the planning and delivery of nursing services for the plastic surgery patient.

Measurement Criteria:

The plastic surgery nurse:

- Evaluates factors related to safety, effectiveness, availability, cost and benefits, efficiencies, and impact on practice when choosing among plastic surgery practice options that would result in the same expected outcome.

- Helps the plastic surgery patient and family in identifying and obtaining appropriate and available services to address health-related needs.

- Assigns or delegates tasks, based on the needs and condition of the plastic surgery patient and family, potential for harm, stability of the patient's condition, complexity of the task, and predictability of the outcome.

- Assists the plastic surgery patient and family in becoming informed consumers about the options, costs, risks, and benefits of treatment and care.

Additional Measurement Criteria for the Advanced Practice Registered Nurse:

The advanced practice registered nurse in plastic surgery:

- Utilizes organizational and community resources to formulate multidisciplinary or interdisciplinary plans of care for the plastic surgery patient.

- Develops creative solutions for problems in plastic surgery patient care that address effective resource utilization and maintenance of quality.

- Develops evaluation strategies to demonstrate cost effectiveness, cost benefit, and efficiency factors associated with nursing practice for the plastic surgery patient.

The content in this appendix is not current and is of historical significance only.

STANDARD 15. LEADERSHIP

The plastic surgery nurse provides leadership in the professional practice setting and the profession.

Measurement Criteria:

The plastic surgery nurse:

- Engages in teamwork as a team player and a team builder.

- Works to create and maintain healthy work environments in local, regional, national, or international communities.

- Displays the ability to define a clear vision, the associated goals, and a plan to implement and measure progress.

- Demonstrates a commitment to continuous, lifelong learning for self and others.

- Teaches others to succeed by mentoring and other strategies.

- Exhibits creativity and flexibility through times of change.

- Demonstrates energy, excitement, and a passion for quality work.

- Willingly accepts mistakes by self and others, thereby creating a culture in which risk-taking is not only safe, but expected.

- Encourages loyalty by valuing people as the most precious asset in an organization.

- Directs the coordination of care across settings and among caregivers, including supervision of licensed and unlicensed personnel in any assigned or delegated tasks as appropriate.

- Serves in important roles in the work setting by participating on committees, councils, and administrative teams.

- Promotes advancement of the profession through participation in professional organizations, such as the American Society of Plastic Surgical Nurses.

Additional Measurement Criteria for the Advanced Practice Registered Nurse:

The advanced practice registered nurse:

- Works to influence decision-making bodies to improve care for the plastic surgery patient.

The content in this appendix is not current and is of historical significance only.

- Provides direction to enhance the effectiveness of the healthcare team.

- Initiates and revises protocols or guidelines to reflect evidence-based practice, to reflect accepted changes in care management for the plastic surgery patient, or to address emerging problems.

- Promotes communication of information and advancement of the profession through writing, publishing, and presentations for professional or lay audiences.

- Designs innovations to effect change in practice and improve health outcomes.

The content in this appendix is not current and is of historical significance only.

GLOSSARY

Criteria. Relevant, measurable indicators of the standards of clinical nursing practice.

Healthcare team. A set of individuals with special expertise who provide healthcare services or assistance to patients. They may include nurses, physicians, psychologists, social workers, nutritionists/dieticians, and various therapists. Healthcare providers also may include service organizations and vendors. A team is comprised of a number of persons associated together in work or activity.

Holism (holistic). A view of everything in terms of patterns and processes that combine to form a whole, instead of seeing things as fragments, pieces, or parts. Holistic nursing embraces nursing practice, which has healing the whole person as its goal. Holism involves understanding the individual as an integrated whole interacting with and being acted upon by both internal and external environments.

Interdisciplinary. Reliant on the overlapping skills and knowledge of each team member and discipline, resulting in synergistic effects where outcomes are enhanced and more comprehensive than the simple aggregation of any team member's individual efforts.

Multidisciplinary. Relating to, or using a combination of, several disciplines for a common purpose. A multidisciplinary team is a unit composed of individuals with varied and specialized expertise who coordinate their activities to provide services to patients with an actual or potential diagnosis. The team engages in collaborative endeavors using the combined skills and expertise of team members. The patent is a member of the team whenever possible and appropriate.

Role. A function. The characteristic and expected social behavior of an individual in relationship to a group.

Standard. An authoritative statement enunciated and promulgated by the profession, by which the quality of practice, service, or education can be judged.

The content in this appendix is not current and is of historical significance only.

REFERENCES

American Board of Medical Specialties. 2000. *Member Boards and Associate Members.* http://www.abms.org/member.asp (accessed February 16, 2004).

American Board of Plastic Surgery. 2003. *About ABPS.* http://www.abplsurg.org/about_abps.html#Description%20of%20Plastic%20Surgery (accessed February 20, 2004).

American Nurses Association. 1995. Committee on Nursing Practices and Guidelines. *Manual to develop guidelines.* Washington, DC: American Nurses Association.

———. 2000. *Scope and standards of practice for nursing professional development.* Washington, DC: nursebooks.org.

———. 2001. *Code of ethics for nurses with interpretive statements.* Washington, DC: ANA.

———. 2003. *Nursing's social policy statement,* 2nd edition. Washington, DC: ANA.

———. 2004. *Nursing: Scope and standards of practice.* Washington, DC: ANA.

American Society of Plastic and Reconstructive Surgical Nurses. 2002. *About ASPSN.* http://www.aspsn.org/ABOUT/objectives.html (accessed March 16, 2004).

American Society of Plastic Surgeons. 2004. *Procedural statistics trends 1992–2003.* http://www.plasticsurgery.org/public_education/Statistical-Trends.cfm (accessed March 16, 2004).

The content in this appendix is not current and is of historical significance only.

BIBLIOGRAPHY

American Society of Plastic and Reconstructive Surgical Nurses. 1987. *Standards for plastic surgical nurses.* Pitman, NJ: ASPRSN.

———. 1996. *Standards for plastic surgical nurses,* 2nd edition. Pitman, NJ: ASPRSN.

———. 1996. *Core curriculum for plastic and reconstructive surgical nursing,* 2nd edition. Pitman, NJ: American Society of Plastic Surgical Nurses.

Association of periOperative Registered Nurses. 2001. *Standards, recommended practices and guidelines.* Denver, CO: AORN.

Brunner, L., and Suddarth, D. 2000. *Textbook of medical surgical nursing.* Philadelphia: Lippincott.

Carpenito, L. 2004. *Nursing diagnosis: Application to clinical practice.* Philadelphia: Lippincott.

Dermatology Nurses Association. 2002. *Dermatology nursing scope of practice and dermatology nursing standards of clinical practice.* Pitman, NJ: DNA.

Goodman, T., ed. 1988. *Core curriculum for plastic and reconstructive surgical nursing.* Pitman, NJ: American Society of Plastic Surgical Nurses.

Index

Note: Entries with [2005] indicate an entry from *Plastic Surgery Nursing: Scope and Standards of Practice* (2005), reproduced in Appendix A. That information is not current but included for historical value only.

A

AAAASF. *See* American Association for Accreditation of Ambulatory Surgery Facilities, Inc. (AAAASF)

AAAHC. *See* Accreditation Association for Ambulatory Health Care (AAAHC)

AAAHC Institute for Quality Improvement (IQI), 13, 68, 70

Abilities in plastic surgery nursing practice, 8, 12
   See also Knowledge, skills, abilities, and judgment

ABMS. *See* American Board of Medical Specialties (ABMS)

ABPS. *See* American Board of Plastic Surgery (ABPS)

Accountability in plastic surgery nursing practice
   aesthetic nurse, 15
   leadership and, 42
   quality of practice and, 39, 89

Accreditation Association for Ambulatory Health Care (AAAHC), 13, 68, 70

Advanced practice registered nurses (APRNs) in plastic surgery nursing practice, 8, 64
   assessment competencies, 20
      measurement criteria [2005], 75–76
   collaboration competencies, 44–45
      measurement criteria [2005], 95–96
   collegiality competencies
      measurement criteria [2005], 93–94
   consultation competencies, 30
      measurement criteria [2005], 85
   coordination of care competencies, 27
      measurement criteria [2005], 83
   diagnosis competencies, 21
      measurement criteria [2005], 77
   education competencies, 37
      measurement criteria [2005], 91
   environmental health competencies, 48
   ethics competencies, 35
      measurement criteria [2005], 97
   evaluation competencies, 32–33
      measurement criteria [2005], 87–88

Expected outcomes in plastic surgery
nursing practice
diagnosis and, 21, 77
evaluation and, 32, 87
outcomes identification and, 22, 78, 79
planning and, 23, 80
See also Evaluation; Outcomes
identification; Planning

F

Families and plastic surgery nursing
practice, 5, 10, 12, 18, 25, 29, 33, 41,
43, 44, 48, 58, 59, 62, 67, 71
See also Healthcare consumers

Financial issues. *See* Cost and economic
controls

Follow-up care in plastic surgery nursing
practice, 14, 15, 16, 69, 70

Foundation of plastic surgery nursing
practice, 1–2
[2005], 58–59

H

Health Insurance Portability and
Accountability Act (HIPAA), 12,
68, 75

Health teaching and promotion in plastic
surgery nursing practice
competencies involving, 28–29
Standard of Practice, 28–29
[2005], 84

Healthcare consumers in plastic surgery
nursing practice, 5–6
aesthetic plastic surgery population,
6–7
reconstructive plastic surgery
population, 6
[2005], 71–72
well-being, 16, 72
See also Families

Healthcare team in plastic surgery
nursing practice, 49
[2005] defined, 102

HIPAA. *See* Health Insurance Portability
and Accountability Act (HIPAA)

Holism (holistic nursing) in plastic
surgery nursing practice, 49
[2005] defined, 102

Hospital environment in plastic surgery
nursing practice, 13
[2005], 68

I

Implementation in plastic surgery
nursing practice
competencies involving, 25–26
Standard of Practice,
25–26
[2005], 82

Information in plastic surgery nursing
practice. *See* Data and
information

Insurance reimbursements in plastic
surgery nursing practice, 17–18
[2005], 74

Interdisciplinary teams in plastic surgery
nursing practice [2005], 82, 87, 91,
93, 94, 95, 97, 99
defined, 102

Interprofessional teams in plastic surgery
nursing practice, 3, 9
competencies involving, 24, 27, 35,
39, 41, 42, 43, 44, 47
defined, 49
See also Collaboration

IQI. *See* AAAHC Institute for Quality
Improvement (IQI)

J

Judgment in plastic surgery nursing
practice, 8, 16, 36, 37, 43,
65, 72
See also Knowledge, skills, abilities,
and judgment

K

Knowledge, skills, abilities, and judgment in plastic surgery nursing practice, 2, 3, 6, 7, 8, 10, 11, 13, 14
  assessment competencies, 19, 20
  collaboration competencies, 44
  education competencies, 36, 37
  environmental health competencies, 48
  evidence-based practice and research competencies, 38
  implementation competencies, 25, 26
  leadership competencies, 43
  planning competencies, 24
  prescriptive authority and treatment competencies, 31
  See also Critical thinking; Education; Evidence-based practice (EBP) and research

L

Laser resurfacing, 5

Laws and regulations in plastic surgery nursing practice, 8, 31, 69, 70, 80, 86, 87

Leadership in plastic surgery nursing practice
  competencies involving, 42–43
  Standard of Professional Performance, 42–43
    [2005], 100–101

M

Measurement criteria. *See* Criteria

Media coverage in plastic surgery nursing practice, 2, 58, 63
  See also Advertising, misleading

Medical errors, 41

Medical spas, plastic surgery nursing practice, 15–16

Multidisciplinary team of plastic surgery nursing practice, 4, 60, 66, 83, 89, 99
  [2005] defined, 102

N

National Federation for Specialty Nursing Organizations, 4, 61

National Institute of Nursing Research (NINR), 61

National Specialty Nursing Certifying Organization (NSNCO), 63

NINR. *See* National Institute of Nursing Research (NINR)

NP. *See* Nurse practitioner (NP)

NSNCO. *See* National Specialty Nursing Certifying Organization (NSNCO)

Nurse practitioner (NP), 8, 64

Nursesbooks.org, vi

Nursing: Scope and Standards of Practice, Second Edition, 7

Nursing care. *See* Care and caring

Nursing competence. *See* Competencies

Nursing education. *See* Education

Nursing judgment. *See* Knowledge, skills, abilities, and judgment in plastic surgery nursing practice

Nursing standards. *See* Standards of Practice; Standards of Professional Performance

Nursing's Social Policy Statement, 62

Nursing's Social Policy Statement: The Essence of the Profession, 7

O

Occupational Safety and Health Administration (OSHA), 13, 69

Office-based surgery centers in plastic surgery nursing practice, 14
  [2005], 69–70

Operative stage of plastic surgery procedure, 2, 13, 14, 59, 66, 68, 70

OSHA. *See* Occupational Safety and Health Administration (OSHA)